MW00953221

Cane Confessions

The Lighter Side to Mobility

Amy L. Bovaird

Copyright © 2016 Amy Bovaird
Copyright © 2016 Cover Image Bernadette Harrison
Copyright © 2016 Cover Production Heather Desuta
Published by Ant Press, 2016

The author asserts the moral right under the Copyright, Designs and Patents Act 1988 to be identified as the author of this work.

All rights reserved. No part of this publication may be reproduced, stored in a retrieval system, or transmitted, in any form or by any means without the prior written consent of the author, nor be otherwise circulated in any form of binding or cover other than that in which it is published and without a similar condition being imposed on the subsequent purchaser.

This book is nonfiction, based on events in the author's life. The names of characters, except for family members, have been changed to protect the privacy of each individual. Place names have, for the most part, been retained because they deserve high recognition for their excellence.

For Aldine Hecker.
Happy ninety-first birthday!
Thank you for believing my stories can have an impact on people.

CONTENTS

INTRODUCTION

I happened to be selling my first book at a craft show not long after it came out. A young woman came up to the table, and I saw her through a smoky haze. After greeting her cheerfully, I asked, "Do you know anyone who is vision-impaired?"

There was a short pause. Then she said, "Yes."

Happy to have found common ground, I asked, "Who?" I was looking for some kind of relationship—a cousin, a friend or even a sibling.

She replied, "You."

"Me! Oh. Sorry, umm, I didn't see…I mean…I didn't know…what I'm trying to say is, I couldn't…." I stopped explaining. The laughter bubbled out of me when I finally recognized Leslie, a family friend.

That hit close to home.

If you're losing your vision, maybe the stories that follow will hit close to home. I hope they do. You may have even had similar tactics and responses in many incidents. If your vision is good, I hope the insights in my stories will help you see me more clearly. I trust they will bring you closer to understanding the challenges a vision-impaired person goes through and cause you to reach out.

I had lived the life of a gypsy, teaching English as a second language and traveling around the world, even after I was diagnosed with an incurable genetic eye disease and told I would go blind—hoping then to burn memories for when I could no longer see. Surprisingly, my eyesight remained relatively stable, allowing me to continue my life of adventure.

Decades later, I returned home after my father was diagnosed with Stage-4 cancer and passed away. Divorced, I moved back to northwest Pennsylvania permanently. Coming home turned into more of a transition than recovering from the loss of my father. My eyesight rapidly deteriorated and catapulted me into another type of "foreign" country— one without many visual cues. I scrambled for help in order to retain my teaching jobs. It became a crossroads period in my life and the subject of my first book, *Mobility Matters: Stepping Out in Faith.*

Four years ago, my vision loss worsened to the point I couldn't manage my classroom anymore and I retired. I turned to writing and began to reinvent myself, using my writing as a vehicle to encourage, inspire and educate others about the world of vision loss.

Since my vision often played tricks on me (my way of saying it was unreliable), life was pretty adventuresome. I had lived in several foreign

1

countries, and using a cane felt foreign to me too. "It's a tool, and you use it when you need it," my trainer said. "But carry it with you all the time, because you never know when you'll need it." His words boxed me in at first. The challenge was to get past the fear "that stick" would rob me of my independence. Or the way people viewed me would steal my capabilities. Trusting my cane has been a process. It's not a perfect solution—as you will see—but it helps me every day and, for that, I'm full of gratitude.

The other tool that enables me to maneuver around my obstacles is the humor arising from my daily life. I feel a sense of comedic action—like I've stepped into Lucille Ball's or Jerry Lewis's shoes at times—but it's my feet making all the moves.

It's a big relief to share—call it a confession of sorts—the situations I faced before I had my cane, the discoveries I made transitioning to use it and after, when I was more comfortable. Losing one's vision isn't so dark and gloomy. It's time to sweep on over to the lighter side of mobility.

To those losing their vision from Retinitis Pigmentosa (RP for short) or to any of my vision-impaired colleagues, search for the good. Whether you attach a pencil tip to your cane—the better to write your experiences down—or a rollerball tip—roll on by the bad.

Whatever you're coping with today, you have an awesome walking stick as well. Hold it upright, move it forward, navigate around the obstacles, explore your environment. Do seek out the positive. Don't be afraid to confess—I mean, share—your stories.

Walk with your head high and let the sunshine wash over you. Let faith and laughter accompany you to maintain the right perspective each day.

1/ SWEET OILS OF DENIAL

Helen, Roberta, Anne and I each went to Manaltheeram, an Ayurvedic spa in South India, for different treatments. Helen suffered from rheumatoid arthritis. Roberta wanted to rejuvenate her skin. Anne had tricky knees, and I, poor vision.

The spa took a holistic approach to health, with the doctor assigning various diets, special oils and massage treatment, all of which cleared the pores. I was told, "You have to start with ridding the toxins from the inside out."

In the mornings, we each went for our separate treatments, and in the early afternoons we girls met up for lunch. I loved the food, so different to my usual palate—vegetarian curries, leafy soups, basmati rice cooked in long green bamboo shoots. Every dish was bathed in distinct coconut sauces.

Later we headed out to sightsee in the local area—to the little shops, to the backwaters or to view traditional dancing. We even met up with a local family Helen knew. Afternoons were lovely.

The problem came in the evenings. Unfortunately, when night fell, so did I. Once when I left a small shop in Kovalam, I stumbled over some loose pebbles and slid into a deep rain gutter. Generally the feeble lighting didn't extend beyond the dim interior of the hole-in-the-wall tourist traps. Not many street lights existed.

At my cry for help, a surprised shopkeeper threw the heavy curtain to his shop open and raced to the rescue, pulling me out of the ditch and brushing me off. The girls followed close behind him. I had worn a long skirt, and one of my companions pointed out the fall had caused a big tear in the material.

The shopkeeper's hands fluttered back and forth as if my fall had shocked him. Maybe he thought an injured tourist would cause him trouble.

This fall—my worst yet—forced me to come clean with the girls about losing my vision. "I hope this treatment helps my eyes," I tried to joke, "Otherwise the landscape is going to do me in."

"We didn't know," Helen said.

"You should have said something," Roberta echoed.

"It's not that big a deal," I murmured, wincing at the bruises. "We all have something...."

By the fourth day, I had become accustomed to our routine and particularly liked our trained masseuses: Lalan, a petite-boned, delicate woman, and Aditi, the larger and younger of the two. Sometimes they took turns, and other times they worked together.

That day, Lalan had just finished up with my massage treatment. The slender Hindu woman handed me a towel to wrap around my hair. Her thick braid fell forward as she gathered up a collection of odd-shaped brown and blue bottles filled with various oils. She blew out the flickering flame then squeezed the wick between her thumb and forefinger to ensure it was out before tucking the candle into a brown wicker bag.

As I wound the towel around my hair, I watched her swish a small hand towel over the stone floor with her bare foot and expertly toss it up a few inches to catch it in one hand. *How did she do that?*

"Thank you, Lalan." I handed her five crisp bills as a tip. She tucked the rupees into the bodice of her indigo-blue sari. She brought her hands together and slid them down to her heart, bowing slightly.

"Lalan, the thatched kiosk by the sea tomorrow?"

"Yes, Madame, if it's available."

How I hoped it was! Gentle breezes moved the fronds of nearby coconut palms that lined the beach. Waves intermittently lapped at the shoreline. Though the idyllic view appeared somewhat blurry to me, the sounds of the relaxing environment were enough to lull me into a light sleep. At a higher elevation, that treatment room was the best at the spa.

I put on my sunglasses, an essential protection against the bright Indian sun, and tied my robe more tightly before easing my feet into the cheap green thongs. Hopefully I would make it back to my cottage before the footwear fell off. Not only were they a one-size-fits-all, but the massage oils made my feet slippery too.

When I first arrived, it seemed strange to walk around the Ayurvedic spa wearing only a green robe and flimsy bath shoes with a towel coiled around my head like a turban. But when I saw how many others—Indians and western patients alike—wandered across the grounds and dined in the open-air cafés in the same attire, I stopped feeling self-conscious. In fact, it was one of the nicer quirks about staying in South India.

After the relaxing, hot oil body massage, I headed back to my cottage—a cute stone and thatched-roof bungalow surrounded by palm trees—slip-sliding on the pathway stones in my floppy thongs. Strains of music wafted in the breeze.

I spotted a tall, Indian man wearing blue jeans, a bright-colored dress shirt and dark shades. Walking backward, he crooned into a microphone. As I moved closer, I saw another man following him with a video recorder. Intrigued, I stopped to watch. They didn't look like ordinary people or even tourists, and Manaltheeram wasn't any ordinary setting.

With palm trees gently swaying in the breeze, a thick carpet of green grass covering the ground, round tables in the open-air café to the left of the men and the picturesque cottages to the right, the landscape looked stunning. The gray sky held only a few low clouds and seemed to reach down to touch the sudsy waves below. Though it was the rainy season, it seemed like we might escape any imminent downpour.

Edging closer—just about ten feet away—I could see the singer's shirt was unbuttoned halfway down to his waist. He looked boyishly charming, though he was probably in his forties. I had no idea which language he was using—Tamil, Hindi or Malayalam, the local dialect of Kerala—but it sounded like the distinct melody of a love song. The singer stopped briefly to confer with the videographer, then he started up again.

Suddenly, a third man came out from who-knew-where to blot and powder the star's face. *Who is this singer? He must be famous!* I stared from the pathway, fascinated. The make-up man darted from view. The singer started singing again, holding the microphone nonchalantly, moving with the kind of swagger that comes from knowing one has charisma.

I needed to return home, but they were right next to the green hammock in front of my cottage. How could I get there without interrupting the film shoot? I contemplated briefly, remembering there was a second path home from the Ayurvedic center. It took me directly behind my cottage, so I could bypass the group.

As I retraced my steps, the strains of music grew fainter. The path veered to a "Y" and I followed it out, toes gripping tightly at the rubber thongs, thinking how good it would be to take a tepid shower. Then I would meet up with the girls for a delicious meal, keeping within the dietary boundaries assigned to me. Everything on the menu tasted light and fresh.

With my mind on brunch, I continued to make my way home. When I looked up, I couldn't believe my eyes! Had I somehow crossed onto the earlier path? Had my eyes played yet another trick on me? How had this happened?

I found myself between the singer and his producer. The filming stopped.

If I had continued a single step farther, I would have fallen headlong into the star, but I caught myself just in time. A few seconds passed without a word. We all stood motionless.

I shifted and regained my balance. What else could the poor man do except burst out laughing? I'm sure I looked pitiful clutching my baggy robe, my white tote hanging limply in the other hand. My head towel hung down on one side, and my hair probably looked as if it had been hot oil-glued to my head. I reeked of a strange odor—a combination of papaya, coconut oil and the special treatment herbs for my vision.

5

Bringing my hands together in the same prayer-like manner Lalan had shown me earlier, I lowered my hands and bowed slightly.

"Namaste," I said, trying to keep a straight face.

The singer looked at me in amusement and smiled. "Hello, Miss!" he returned in English. His cameraman did not smile. The singer refrained from shaking my hand, which was a relief as it, too, was covered in a film of oil.

A woman appeared with dark, wavy hair falling loosely over her shoulders. She was dressed in the typical, fitted midriff blouse in electric blue over a bright yellow sari and wore dark high heels. When she glanced my way, I noticed an elegant blue *bindi* between her eyebrows and dark sunglasses perched on her head. The beautiful woman spoke quickly. I couldn't detect which dialect she used, but I could tell by the way she started waving her sunglasses around she was not pleased. The singer smiled my way and shrugged his shoulders comically, not in the least put out.

"So sorry, I…um…." The next few words sat still on my tongue, but my lips continued to move like a fish gasping for air. Filling in the blanks with "got lost," would have sounded like the weakest trick in the book to gain access to a celebrity—something Lucille Ball might have resorted to. And here I was imitating her antics—but in real life.

Finally, I pointed. "That's my cottage." Everyone turned to look at it, as if on cue. I imagined the singer breaking out in song, gesturing to my cozy cottage and then to me and ad-libbing a few lines. My heart swelled in excitement. But the spell broke. The woman arranged her matching electric blue *dupatta* over her shoulders and never looked my way again. To her I was simply an intrusion, a wide-eyed, slicked-down, green-robed, smelly westerner who dared to interrupt a star's photoshoot.

The video producer gestured to the star for a quick touch-up and waved the woman away. Was she a star, too? A singer? The girlfriend? Their break was over, and it was time to resume filming.

I took my cue and scuttled up the stairs to my cottage. Instead of taking my typical late morning shower, I couldn't resist peeking out the window at their progress. Later, people told me the singer was a famous movie star in Kerala and that many such stars came to Manaltheeram to film on location.

I never quite figured out what caused me to land directly in front of the singer; whether I took the same footpath twice or remembered incorrectly, I never found out. While the incident amused me, I couldn't help but think back to the words of my eye specialist about fifteen years earlier. "You will go blind. I don't know when. It could be tomorrow, in five years or sometime down the line. The only certainty is that your condition is progressive, so it *will* happen."

Although I had gone to South India for holistic treatment in improving my eyes, I had to face the truth—my condition had progressed. Retinitis Pigmentosa (RP) was robbing my sight so gradually that degrees of denial had set in, like the layers of oil that covered my skin. I slipped from year to year without paying much attention. I never took the time to analyze what was happening. Instead, I adjusted to the situation, going full speed ahead to each new pathway. That's how I held myself together emotionally.

In India, the abrupt shift from light to darkness halted me once the sun went down. Had I been monitoring and accepting the progress of my RP, I might have been using a cane. As it was, I simply took the arm of one of the girls to help me find my way. But during daylight hours, it was easier to wash away the fear as I splashed in the sunny water of travel. Slip-sliding through RP had become my way of life.

2/ HOW I BECAME A ROYAL PAIN

Before I used a cane, I depended on my faulty eyes to get me where I needed to be. I have to confess that, without my cane sidekick, life challenged me. Still, I never imagined I had a choice or a more dependable way of making sure I arrived without a trail of shocked eyes following. Such was the case when I greeted royalty in the United Arab Emirates.

As a new language instructor at a women's college, I quickly learned about Arab customs and the fascinating world of sheikhs—Arab royalty. Each emirate had its own royal family and entourage.

Before classes started, the college system I belonged to kicked off the academic year with a large conference in the capital, Abu Dhabi. I lived in Ras Al Khaimah—informally called RAK—two and a half hours to the north. The name, translated, means "Head of the Tent."

In the early morning darkness, the teachers of the men and women's colleges strapped themselves into the hard fiberglass seats of an old military seaplane. Ed, the lone director of both colleges, reminded me of a low-key general, with his lanky height and easy smile. He was the last to take his seat.

"Now remember, all new faculty members will meet the Chancellor of our college system. This is a great honor and your chance to shine." He shook a finger at us. "Don't screw around. You're representing *me* out there. We may be from the desert, but we're no country bumpkins."

That year, we had an unusually high number of new hires as well as the old teachers on board, all looking forward to the big day in the city, away from the goats and camels.

Hundreds of beaming faculty members from around the country congregated in a fancy Abu Dhabi hotel every year. Between speeches, the teachers networked with each other at informal meet-and-greets. I recall looking across the length of the polished tiles and seeing a mixture of international and Emirati faculty reaching for heavy water goblets, sipping from tea cups and nibbling date cookies on silver platters.

My colleagues awed me. They all had smiles on their faces and name tags clipped to their shirts or collars. Some slung conference bags over their shoulders or snapped open briefcases as they reached for their name cards.

The local women stood in clusters with their black *sheylas* covering their hair and floor-length *abiyahs*, revealing an occasional colorful peek at their dresses underneath. The local men wore white or checkered *ghutras* hanging from their heads and ambled comfortably in their customary white *dishdashas* and sandals. The heavy sweet perfume, which I later learned was Oud, clung to the folds of fabric around me on both men and women. However, not everyone dressed in traditional attire. Some of the locals wore western suits.

As we broke for lunch, my friend, Carol, jabbed me in the side. "Look at those tables!"

My eyes took in the enormous buffet laden with Middle Eastern cuisine. My stomach growled. "Come on, let's get in line."

From living in Egypt, I recognized a few of the salads like *hummus* and *baba ganoush*—more of what westerners would call dips—along with the bowls of toasted triangles from the pita-like bread next to them. The fragrant soups tempted me. I ladled out a cup of the thick lentil soup, spilling some on the white linen tablecloth as I missed the bowl. *Oh! Napkin!* I searched frantically, but found nothing. Carol stepped out of line and returned with a cloth napkin.

"It's all I could find," she apologized as she helped me mop it up.

"Thank you," I mouthed. Quickly moving on, I served myself some of the finger food, tightly-wrapped Lebanese stuffed grape leaves and *halwa*, squares made from sesame paste.

I paused, knowing that if I tried to carry any more food, I risked dropping my bowl and plate. Even carrying this had its risks.

"Let me get that," Carol offered. She knew how hard I had to focus to find my way back to my seat. Gratefully, I handed her my dishes.

As we went through the next line, we found trays of savory foods, others that wafted several pungent Indian spices, and then sweet dishes. We encountered every kind of meat imaginable, but I dished up only a few to sample. My eyes were often bigger than my stomach. As we left, I tramped on the woman's heel ahead of me.

"Sorry! 'Scuse me," I yelped, stricken. "I didn't see you...."

Half an hour later, completely full, I dabbed my mouth with a cloth napkin.

"I don't even want to think about dessert," I croaked, still letting my eyes roam to the dessert table. On one end, I glimpsed a favorite of mine: *basbousa*, its wafer-thin layers dripping in syrup, followed by several small, pretty tea cakes. Then a large silver container I knew held *Om Ali*—Egyptian bread pudding.

"No one can pass these up," Carol agreed, and we stood in that line too.

Soon it would be time for the big event.

Like all the new hires, I could hardly wait to meet the Chancellor— probably the most celebrated sheikh in the country—and his entourage.

Each director led his or her new flock to a special receiving room to wait in line for the honor of shaking his hand. We were briefed on the protocol. The director would formally introduce each faculty member. We would take his hand, shake once and move on.

That seemed easy enough.

The procession started. I was carrying a bulky present to give to a friend who worked in the Abu Dhabi campus, but I hadn't found her yet. I tried to pawn it off on a teacher with a bigger purse. As we went forward, I desperately tried to get her attention. She leaned toward me, distracted, "Sorry dear, what do you want?"

She politely smiled and turned away, as if she hadn't heard my request. She, too, was focused on her moment with the sheikh.

I started to panic. What was I going to do with it when I had to shake hands?

Blasted! Me and my gift-giving dilemmas. Did this happen to anyone else? I sincerely doubted it. I never imagined it would take me so long to locate my friend. But I never dreamed we would have a crowd this size either.

With the quietest of feet, we crossed over a plush, carpeted area in the hotel. The room took on a hushed tone of formality. My heart beat faster. In the next room, I would come face-to-face—rather, hand-to-hand—with the sheikh.

In a matter of minutes, I'd be facing a line of very important men in silk robes. I inched forward. Stayed in line. The line moved faster and faster. I kept my eyes on the entourage. I didn't want to miss a second of this experience. My heart pounded. Soon it would be my turn.

As I craned my head, I caught a glimpse of the sheikh in his traditional gold *thobe*, looking regal and benevolent as he leaned over to shake each hand.

What was I going to do with the bulky gift?

I put it under my arm, and as I moved forward, it slipped down to my side. Not going to work. What if it fell at the sheikh's feet as I leaned toward him?

Suddenly, my eyesight blurred. Every once in a while, my vision fogged up out of the blue. When this happened, I blinked, trying to get the images back. But usually the opposite happened, the details in my line of sight disappeared, selectively so; this meant I could see some things but not others. I could see the carpet, the walls and parts of the furniture, but I couldn't see Ed, my presenter. I knew he was there somewhere, but it was like looking at air.

Oh no! I frantically sought out Ed's lanky form. I had to find him. Now! My breath started coming faster. Where was he? I turned from side to side. No Ed. Meanwhile, I continued to move forward, so focused on keeping up in the procession without tripping over whomever I might not see that I completely forgot about the bulky parcel I was carrying. I kept walking forward.

Until....

"Whoa!" Ed's astonished voice was so close that it startled me. "You passed right by the sheikh!"

I gasped.

Ed deftly looped me around for the introduction, which made everyone else who followed me in line, stop.

"Amy Bovaird, English faculty member from America," Ed announced as we reached the sheikh.

This is it!

At Ed's nudge, I reached out with clammy, trembling fingers and took the sheikh's hand. It wasn't until our hands touched that I realized something felt wrong—out of place. And no wonder. I had reached out with my free hand, the *left* one.

After the perfunctory shake, I pulled my hand back as if I had touched something hot. Ed's stiff-lipped, shocked expression told me he had witnessed my blunder. Blunder? Was there even a word big enough for what I had done?

I just took the sheikh's hand with what the Arab world consider to be the *toilet* hand.

The line behind me moved forward. I heard Ed announce the next honoree to the prestigious sheikh as I moved forward to greet the entourage in a daze. I snapped out of my trance and freed my right hand to shake their hands, barely touching the tips of their fingers with my own. My heart beat out a repetitive tune of I-can't-believe-I-did-that.

It all happened so fast. I felt the heat of my embarrassment start at the roots of my hair and travel to my face, down my neck. I'm sure it didn't stop until it reached my toes. My stomach churned and my chest heaved up and down in disbelief. I felt sick to my stomach as I reached the edge of the soft carpet and headed down the marble steps.

I wasn't a newbie to the Arab culture. This wasn't my first encounter in the Middle East by a long shot. I had taught English to Saudis, Egyptians, Pakistanis, Moroccans, Tunisians—and many others—for years. Arab Culture 101: Never extend your left hand to another person, because it's dirty. Parents model this to their children even before they can speak, regardless of their social status. It is *haram*—forbidden—in all circles in every Arab culture around the world.

I groaned and shook my hand as if it were, indeed, *dirty*. I could hardly breathe as I relived the moment in slow motion...a blunder with the most prestigious man in the country.

What must the sheikh have thought? Did he wipe his hand on his *thobe* the moment he had the opportunity? He probably rushed off to the bathroom to wash it the instant the procession finished. Oh no! The sheikh knew my name! Would I get fired? What would I tell them back home? "Yeah, it didn't work out. You see, I had a dirty hand." I cringed. What would I say to the director...or to anyone else? Everyone saw anyway. How could I ever live this down?

But I somehow *did* overcome the embarrassment of that day, and now it makes me laugh. Awkward as it was, I don't believe the sheikh with all his education about western practices believed my hand was dirty or that I was trying to insult him. He probably thought I was a knucklehead or a daydreamer. I'm sure it never entered his head that I was a legally-blind teacher whose vision played tricks on her and who should have had a cane.

Though I never found out what the Chancellor thought about my ill-fated greeting, I'd like to think he was the kind of sheikh who wouldn't get all shook up over the wrong hand shake.

3/ SEPARATING THE KIDS FROM THE GOATS

Having low vision and a penchant for stumbling, I shouldn't have been kidding around on any kind of mountain called Goatfell. My mother has often said I'm so stubborn it's downright bothersome. I'm like a goat myself, bucking good sense and bleating non-stop about it.

From Ardrossan, Scotland, a short trip by ferry carries passengers to the largest island in the Firth of Clyde. Scots call it the Isle of Arran, rolling their r's in a cozy way. I rubbed my hands together. I couldn't wait to get off the ferry and explore. Luckily, I met a middle-aged couple eager to extol the island's charms to a traveler.

"Arran 'tis a scenic place to see. Ye made a good choice there, ye did."

"Aye, so she did," his wife agreed.

The lady, a plump woman in a powder blue raincoat, braced herself against a sudden, fierce gust of wind. She smiled, shielding her eyes from the strands of dark hair that whipped about and escaped from under her scarf.

"Are ye just planning where to go now?" she asked.

"No better time." I liked to think of myself as a flying-by-the-seat-of-my-pants kind of gal. "Are you from Arran? Do you have any recommendations?"

"No, but Robert's family is. We can tell ye a fair number 'a places to see if ye'd like."

"That'd be great!" I took out my pencil and notebook and leaned forward to better decipher their Scottish brogue.

"Brodick has a castle, but ye can see that later," Robert began. "Now Goatfell, the highest peak on Arran, 'tis magnificent and one ye'll not be wantin' to miss."

"Oh no. 'Tis your best bet for today. Not such a hard climb if the weather holds," Ginny agreed.

"'Twill be a good challenge though. Goatfell is what we Scots call a 'Corbett,' a very high mountain ranging from, say...what would it be, Ginny?"

His wife pushed the strands of hair away from her eyes. "Mebbe from 700 to 800 meters."

"Aye. With a slope about...would ye say 90 meters, Ginny?"

"That sounds about right, Robert. So it does."

"Ye can see it from the ferry." Robert pointed to the craggy summit of Goatfell. As a recreational hiker, I had few international climbs to compare it to. It was difficult to anticipate what the journey might entail. But it seemed like a good way to pass the afternoon.

We pulled into the harbor. After a quick thank you to the couple for their help, I waved goodbye, eager to get started.

On foot, the hike to Goatfell took 45 minutes. Of course, asking for directions and frequently shifting the heavy backpack—filled with an entire week's belongings—slowed down the pace. At a convenience store, a pint of milk mixed with some protein powder packed for the journey, provided a boost in energy.

Keep going. You'll soon be at the base of Goatfell where your adventure will start. Optimism returned.

The climb up Goatfell started at midday. Seemingly within minutes, several climbers descended, smiling and energetic. It couldn't be that bad. Within the hour, I was re-thinking my logic. The steep grade of loose dirt and rock proved challenging. My brand new, zoom lens camera fell and banged on the rocks. I finally grabbed the strap and pulled the body up, dented but still operable.

Hiking by road with a monster backpack was nothing compared to lugging it uphill on my shoulders. Other hikers slung small knapsacks over theirs. They didn't seem to mind the steep incline. I huffed and puffed to inhale as much oxygen as possible as they carried on light conversations with one another. They gave each other high fives and downed bottles of spring water while I hadn't the energy to quench my thirst.

Everyday sneakers provided little support for the climb. Others zipped by in sturdy leather hiking boots. As the air became lighter, I had a sneaking (huff!) suspicion I should be heading (huff! puff!) down instead of expending so much energy climbing up the rocky monstrosity.

"H'llo," said a hiker who briefly came abreast. "Masterin' the mighty Corbett, are ye?" In a flash, he passed by, the unuttered response still on my lips.

"The mighty Corbett," I muttered, attempting a stronger foothold in the loose, rocky dirt before taking the next shaky step up. "Whatever happened to that original founding climber? Mountains don't get named after people without them surviving some kind of death-defying odds." Any bet the first Corbett was a Viking?

The fickle Scottish weather played hide-and-seek on the mountain. One minute, the sun blazed down on the path. The next, it snuggled up in the clouds for a short nap so the chill crept in. After being taunted by the elements for too long, I stopped playing the quick-change artist and stored my windbreaker in my sack. At one point, thunder rumbled and splashes of rain pelted the climbers. I longed to fish out my jacket to warm up, but decided against it.

Hikers passed in both directions. No one had a rucksack anywhere near the size of mine. Goatfell meant serious climbing and that meant light loads. But what could I do but limp along, persuading shoulders to do their part along with clumsy feet?

The creek swelled in parts, and water seeped into my shoes. On the slippery path, I had a tough time slogging in my treadless tennis shoes.

Noticing a climber fitted in top-of-the-line hiking attire down to his leather boots, I shouted, "Are those waterproof?" He didn't bother answering the silly question. Of course they were. After that, several hikers, looking dry and fit, filed past, further dampening my morale.

I arched my back in an effort to throw off the fatigue. How much better it would have been to throw off my backpack instead. Bumbling along, I frequently cried out, "Arrgh!" "Ooops!" "Uh-oh!" "Eeeeee–!" "Aaah!" and "'Scuse me!"

Higher up on the trail, an older fellow also seemed to be having his share of obstacles. "Goot a hule in m' shuu," he muttered while plodding on. It took a moment to realize his predicament: a hole in his shoe. If he could go on in spite of his age and difficulties, I could also persevere.

Then the next climber came along. "It gets much worse over the crest." *What? Worse than* this? "It's cloudy, ye canny see anythin' at the top. It's hard to find the pathway, too."

That's all it took. I reached a mental fence that divided the goats from the kids and collapsed.

The end of the line.

I let out a long breath and gulped down a swig of water to get ready for the long trip down Goatfell. "Here we go again," I muttered, bending over to tie a loose shoelace, and started my descent.

The base of Goatfell came into view just as darkness descended. The middle-aged couple ahead of me made plans to stay in the next town over.

"Do you mind if I tag along with you?"

They turned, surprised. They hadn't known a desperate American had latched onto their bright clothing and matched their pace, eavesdropping to boot.

"Sure, come along," the woman invited. "Lord knows we all need fut."

It took me a while to figure what she thought we all needed. Foot? New feet? Hood? Wood—maybe for a fire? Fudge didn't seem far-fetched at that point. Fun? Nearing the restaurant, it became clear—food! So glad they let a stranger tag along since night blindness would have done me in for sure.

Though I didn't have a cane—or even the simpler version, a walking stick—desperation had finally won out and forced me to speak. After that, we shared an evening together over almond-crusted haddock topped with fragrant lemon slices, a goat cheese salad and my first ever fire-lit baked Alaskan dessert. On a full stomach, the bruises seemed less painful.

I have to confess, though making friends is a good reward, spontaneity isn't always my best bet. Starting with ill-suited clothing and the lack of mental preparation, it wasn't exactly the kind of trip I had in mind. The name, Goatfell, should have set off alarm bells. If the goats couldn't climb it without falling, what chance would a vision-impaired gal like me have? I found an altogether new meaning for the term, 'Flying by the seat of my pants.'

The approach I took to climbing the mighty Corbett was often the approach I took to climbing the slippery path of vision loss. Without foresight to plan what tools would best ensure success, I foolishly set out without any and endured various degrees of calamity. Comparing myself and copying what others did never worked for me. I needed my own tools to succeed. While humor helped ease the bruises on my ego, I needed both honesty and a cane to scale farther up beyond the gate that separated the kids from the goats.

Though not quite the triumphant traveler who conquered the mighty Corbett on the Isle of Arran, stubborn determination kept me going. True to nature, I bucked common sense—taking a full-sized backpack up Goatfell—and bleated about this decision up and down the mountain.

While I still struggle with character traits that make even the most stubborn and robust goat susceptible to slipping on Goatfell, I scale higher peaks all the time. I haven't lost the sense of adventure, but now I have the cane and the honesty to go along with it.

I am conquering the mighty Corbett of Vision Loss. How great it will be to follow those who have gone ahead and share a meal of optimism topped with friendly laughter. We'd end it with accepting ourselves exactly as we are. Lord knows, we can all use some of that fut!

4/ BABY STEPS

"Women and Men of Sigma Epsilon Chi, who is ready to participate in Expressions?" The leader of our women's group stood side by side in solidarity with the president of the men's group. "We need 100 percent loyalty in both clubs if we want to take first place! Who's in?"

Hands shot up. Mine too, although normally I'm too shy to speak up and too timid to act. I was like the border of a map, hanging on the fringe of the social club. But that day, something about Sarah's outgoing personality made me want to jump in and participate. I couldn't help but feel it would be fun to join in all the excitement. I vowed to navigate myself more centrally to my club's map.

Loyal? You bet! They'll find a small role just right for me.

Small was right. Or more like...young. Our group sang a song, pitting one generation against the other, and I represented the youngest of the younger generation—a toddler. Holly, our choreographer, thought that role would suit me well.

During our first practice, she stood in a line with us and demonstrated the steps. The second time, we followed her lead. "What are we going to do about the other gen-er-A-tion?" Arm swing and big kick to the right. We practiced that a few times. "What are we going to do about them?" Point to the other group and kick out front.

It seemed so easy until we added more new moves and put them all together. Like line dancers, we linked arms and kicked high. Well, most of us did. I either lagged behind or kicked too early. When I tried to synchronize my steps, watching for the other feet messed me up. I tried a number of ways to keep the right pace. Sometimes I fell in step with the others perfectly, but not always. When we finished singing, "...the other gen-er-A-tion," I kicked hard.

The male voice next to me rose a few octaves. I looked over and saw my Sigma brother bent over double.

"Oww! Whoo-hoo-hoo!" he howled in soprano, giving me a shocked look before limping off the set.

Did I do that? There was no mistaking the destination of the kick. That was painful to watch, let alone know I was responsible for it. How confusing. I had meant to turn in the opposite direction.

The crowd erupted in nervous laughter and whispers. I looked off into space, desperately wanting the moment to pass. When I signed on for the part, I didn't envision such a catastrophe.

At the end of practice, I sought out the choreographer.

"Holly," I said, feeling more like a kindergartener than a college student, "I think I need some extra help with the choreography. I seem to be a bit out of step."

Holly paused and fanned herself with a sheath of papers before giving me a knowing smile. "Ya' think? First of all, we need to move Doug away from you." After a short pause, she said, "You're playing a baby, right?"

"Well, my character is officially listed in the program as a toddler," I said, not sure why I felt I needed to make the distinction.

She ignored the correction. "Real life babies don't get it right either." She clapped her hands. "It doesn't matter if you're out of step with the rest of the cast or not. The whole song is about generations not following each other. So don't worry about it. Oh, and try to remember to kick...low." She smoothed her papers and gave me a bright smile.

Someone else called out, "Holly...."

Pleased she had solved my dilemma so easily, she turned to the voice. "Be right there!"

That wasn't the solution I wanted. It was more like putting a Band-Aid on a scraped knee instead of cleaning the wound so it could heal. But perhaps as long as I kicked low, it would work. So what if I didn't do it perfectly? Babies—or rather toddlers—didn't have to.

The night of the performance, I wore a bonnet and light green flannel footie pajamas. A make-up artist outlined my eyes and colored my cheeks a ruddy red. I put on my own lipstick. The whole get-up looked cute. No one could have smiled more...and probably the audience thought I was purposely out of step. So, as Holly said, it really didn't matter.

I don't remember if Sigma received any awards that night, but my older brother grabbed teasing rights to the lyrics and my choreographed moves. To this day, when he sings, "What are we going to do about the other generation?" and throws himself into it with funny body movements, imitating me, it makes me laugh.

On the one hand, Holly's low expectations of me that night likely contributed to my lax attitude about getting around. On the other, it probably did wonders toward helping me adapt to my changing vision needs. I didn't worry so much about how I looked getting from one place to another as long as I arrived—bruises and all. No wonder I revolted when I met Bob, my mobility instructor.

When it came to mobility training, I experienced the same denial so many others losing their vision face: "I don't need a cane. My vision isn't that bad!" I probably looked on his stick as a chastising tool instead of what it really represented: a more appropriate and safer mobility method. By that time, I was set in my ways. For example, I'd rather walk with my hands moving at various junctures to feel my way than learn how to manipulate a cane and find my obstacles in advance.

I was also terrified of his rhetoric. When he asked me, "Why don't you just tell people you're blind?" I wanted to revert back to my toddler role and block my ears or, better yet, run and hide.

A cane would stifle me, surely hamper my freedom of movement, or so I believed. Worse, what people would think chilled me. People would stare, point and whisper...and, again, I would be an unwanted center of attention.

Yet when I trained with my cane around the neighborhood, bundled in laughter and imagination, I stayed warm, even though I passed through cold and drafty moments of insecurity. The power of positive thinking slipped my arms through the sleeves and zipped up my coat of purpose once more. The coat, padded with down feathers of humor, carried me through that first day.

In subsequent lessons, I donned sleep shades—those black eye coverings some people use to sleep better at night, especially on airplanes—to simulate the conditions I would face in the future. I learned we all live in one world—whether blind or sighted—and the difference is only in the manner in which we perceive the obstacles. One is no less safe or legitimate than the other.

Tangling my cane in a turnstile in one mobility lesson led to a real turn in thinking. I had to push through my fears to develop an evolving mindset about blindness, one that included self-acceptance. That meant I had to strive to overcome any barrier—whatever the turnstile—in living my life the best way possible. Bob also taught me through example to sweep away negative criticism exactly the way I swept my cane back and forth.

Over time, I learned listening for familiar noises or even getting a whiff of coffee bean could help me judge where I was. I discovered how to feel my way around a plate of food so I didn't drop my meal everywhere or knock over my water glass.

Bob taught me how to cross busy intersections, and I finally accepted that when all else failed, it wasn't a disaster to ask someone where I was. Sighted people get lost all the time and probably have fewer qualms about asking for help. Even arranging rides to reach places I couldn't access by myself became a little easier. If a ride didn't pan out in the way I expected, I started making conscious choices to handle the disappointment instead of wallowing in self-pity or anger. In six months, I had the basics down and faced the challenging task of putting the lessons I had learned into practice on my own.

Retracing my steps, I see my biggest hurdle to better mobility was stepping past my *laissez-faire* attitude and overcoming misconceptions about blindness, while coming to terms with my own sight limitations. Both my trust and progress happened in spurts of growth—lots of baby steps. I had to synchronize my thinking with a new way of perceiving my environment. When I talked out the challenges with my mobility instructor, he never simply put Band-Aids on my scraped pride. He worked out real solutions to instill confidence in me.

While I still had several techniques to perfect, I stepped out of my toddler shoes and walked into the active world of mobility.

5/ HOW'S THE VIEW?

Mohamed came into my life at exactly the right time. We met at a Fourth of July picnic hosted by my mobility instructor and Mo was the only person I connected with. We shared an interest in the United Arab Emirates, where we had both lived. Originally from Iraq, Mo had moved to Erie to attend a nearby university for his junior year. Completely blind, Mo not only faced academic challenges, he had to familiarize himself with a new campus—and a fresh major.

The year had been full of massive change for me as I stepped out of my comfort zone and sought help to handle a huge drop in my vision. Since I no longer saw well enough to get around without a cane, I spent six months learning basic mobility techniques. I felt like an adolescent, with an outbreak of pimples and other flaws visible to everyone. My emotions skidded everywhere.

I headed to the Cleveland Sight Center for three weeks of intensive life skills training. My mobility instructor convinced me that not only would I receive the in-depth mobility training I needed, learning other skills would make my life easier. I agreed, but I vacillated between this challenging adventure and being terrified to confront my fears.

Mo and I stayed connected because of our mutual challenges. We each latched onto something the other had. I was an encourager and an educator. Mo, impeded by his blindness, struggled to master the necessary study skills. On the other hand, he had experienced a lifetime of practice dealing with blindness, while I struggled to master both the psychological and physical challenges of my vision loss.

Mo moved on campus in Edinboro the same day I traveled to the Sight Center in Cleveland. As I walked through my efficiency apartment, I thought of Mo settling into his dorm room. I reached for my cell phone.

"Hey, I'm here. How are you settling in?"

"Hi, Grandma, are you an Ohio-ite already? Hey, I'm studying computer science and you are learnin' to be blind."

"I'm not your grandma. And I prefer to say, 'I'm preparing myself to cope with additional vision loss,'" I said crisply.

"Well, you *are* old, more than twice my age." He chuckled. "And what's wrong with sayin' you're learnin' to be blind? That's what you're doing."

His words felt like a bulldozer, smashing what little confidence I'd built. Maybe he was trying to help me see things from another angle.

Maybe he thought he was keeping me grounded in reality. But blindness just happens. It's a condition, not something you learn. I was just learning to cope.

"Where did you pick up 'Ohio-ite?' Your English is really good. You don't even sound like a second language speaker."

"Of course. I prefer English over Arabic."

I walked into the living room and pulled the drawstring to open the venetian blinds. The window overlooked a busy, tree-lined street. "Mo, how do you like the view?"

His silence alerted me to my blunder. I felt so comfortable with Mo, I completely forgot that he couldn't see. "I mean, uh, how do you like your, um, your room?"

"Just like any dorm room," he said, sounding bored. "My roommate doesn't come for another week."

"I don't have a roommate," I teased. "I can do whatever I want."

"Shut up," he said, good-naturedly.

I switched on the television and lowered the volume so I could continue our conversation. "Hey, Mo, have you watched any good movies lately?" I caught myself right away. *What's* wrong *with me? He must think I'm the most insensitive person alive.* "I mean, have you heard any good mo...."

"Grandma, I'm just a regular guy," Mo said with a tinge of impatience. "You don't have to tiptoe around me like the little old lady you are," he added, probably to make me laugh and spare my feelings. "Just speak normally. I know what you mean. You don't have to say, 'hear.' I say I watch movies all the time. When you correct yourself that makes me feel weird and different. Don't do that. Just say what comes to your mind."

"You young whippersnapper. Respect your grandma. I'd better go, though, since I have to get up early." I paused. "Mo, I can do this, right?" I could hear the doubt in my voice.

"Of course you can."

"Thanks. I'll let you know how my training goes tomorrow night."

The next morning, I gathered a sack lunch, my cane and the black sleep shades I would wear for the next eight hours. Slipping the shades over my eyes to prevent me from seeing anything, I opened my cane and left the room. Turning to the left, I swept my way to the end of the corridor. Around the corner, I found the elevator. Inside, I felt for the Braille that would indicate the third floor, the Adjustment to Blindness Wing.

When I pressed the button, static filled the elevator, but it didn't move. Finally, I heard a voice. "Which floor are ya' stuck on?"

That's odd. I didn't hear anyone else in the elevator when I entered.

The voice must be coming from an intercom system. Stuck? The elevator is stuck. Great. My training hasn't even started yet and I'm already having problems. I waved my hand in front of my face to get the air moving and coughed. *Is the heat already pressing in on me? How long before the stalled elevator will be free?*

After a confusing conversation with 'the voice,' where it seemed we were talking at cross purposes, the man exclaimed, "Wait a minute, Ma'am, are you blind?"

"No, no, no." *Was I? I felt as if I were debating a lofty concept with myself. He asked a simple question. Either I was blind or I wasn't. A simple answer would do.* "Yes, I am."

"Now it makes sense. Try pressing the third floor button again."

I felt for the button and pressed. The elevator moved.

"See? Ya' ain't stuck, and neither is this elevator."

"Hooray!"

It turned out when I thought I had pressed the button to the third floor, I must have touched the emergency button instead, calling the maintenance personnel and alerting them to my "situation." After that, we both assumed I was stuck. But the elevator could move perfectly fine.

Even a task as easy as pressing a button became complicated with hampered mobility. I told him how bizarre the whole experience was and apologized for the misunderstanding.

"Wa-al now," the mechanic said, "Ain't no damage done to the elevator, so they's nuthin' to fix. That makes me mighty pleased on a' early Monday mornin', so, lady, I gots to thank ya' for not gettin' stuck in the first place."

I liked the way this man thought. I smiled, imagining him in his cubbyhole office, sipping his coffee. "Hope the rest of your day goes well."

"You, too. It kinda' brightened my morning talking to ya'. Take care, now."

The elevator came to a halt, and the friendly voice disappeared. I shore-lined the wall until I felt the first indentation—a door. I found the knob and turned it. "Hullo. Is this the adjustment to, um, blindness training place?"

"Amy, you made it. It's Betty, the coordinator. Have a seat, five steps in front of you."

By the sounds of the breath she let out when Betty also sat herself down, she was a heavier woman. "Settle down," she said. "We're not going anywhere."

"Thanks. Where were we supposed to…." I stopped.

She chuckled. "Not you. Just telling Charley, my guide dog, to lie down."

Wearing sleep shades made it difficult to tell whom the conversation was directed to. I didn't realize how much eye contact factored into conversations.

Two other adults would be training alongside me, though we all had different goals. We would practice housekeeping, kitchen and meal preparation, Braille and anything that had to do with life skills. The mobility instructor would stop by in the afternoons to take us out to practice one-on-one. We would each work at our own level to improve our skills.

The atmosphere was upbeat. Right away, I heard the clicking of what sounded like an old-fashioned typewriter.

"Betty," a woman who sounded energetic and youthful, called out to the coordinator. "This is a cool recipe. You'd love it. It's got all kinds of healthy ingredients." The rapid clicking continued.

"Is it full of chocolate and nuts? That's what I think a great recipe has." Betty's laughter invited companionship. I liked them both already.

"Amy? I heard you were coming. I'm Luisa. Do you know what a Perkin's Brailler is?"

I shook my head. *Oh, she probably can't see me.* "No," I conceded.

"Come see it," she invited. "Give me your hand."

"It has six keys all together and a center key. See, that one's longer. It's used for spacing. The one on the right is to backspace."

I noticed Luisa used "see" for "feel," and didn't seem at all self-conscious about it. She seemed pretty far along in her Braille. I needed to refresh my skills.

The other trainee arrived. "Hey everyone, I'm here—again." Mark had apparently received training earlier in the year and was continuing on for a second session.

I sat quietly listening to the buzz and busy-ness around me. I looked forward to learning more about my colleagues. Since we were all at different levels, our set-up seemed like a one-room schoolhouse.

Luisa offered, "I heard you have Retinitis Pigmentosa. I do, too. How much can you see? I have almost no vision left."

"I'm completely blind," Mark said, "and I just had a killer year at college, especially traveling from class to class during the winter term. I'll be a sophomore in the fall."

"I can see some, but I'm wearing sleep shades so I can't see anything at the moment." I thought I was brave to wear them. This was their everyday world. It really put what sight I had in perspective.

But neither Mark nor Luisa showed any embarrassment about their degrees of vision loss. The conversation flowed easily between them and the staff. Having never experienced such openness from other people about their vision loss, I found the honesty exhilarating.

Luisa asked me about my cane training. I explained how I had crossed some busy streets and had found my way to the Office of Vocational Rehabilitation after being dropped off in an unknown point in the city.

"Sure, OVR," she said, letting the abbreviation roll off her tongue, demonstrating her familiarity with the system. "I often travel by subway into Pittsburgh. But I want to brush up on my technique to get around more easily," she confided.

I couldn't even imagine how to navigate the subway.

"I'm just trying to make my way down the sidewalk without tripping when I reach a curb," Mark said. "I don't like using a cane. I prefer using a sighted guide on campus, but someone isn't always around to help." He muttered something I couldn't hear. "It's pretty difficult to trust my cane. I wish it would say, 'Snowbank ahead,' or 'Step up, curb.'"

I laughed. "I hear ya'. But we're not far off from when a cane like this will be invented."

How valuable this type of discussion was for someone like me who had never met another person who struggled with vision loss, aside from Mo.

The morning passed quickly. After lunch I heard a new voice.

"Joe's here. Who wants the first mobility lesson?" Luisa called.

Neither Mark nor I spoke up.

"I'll go," Luisa volunteered.

When she returned, Mark took his turn. By the time they came back, it was nearly four o'clock, time for our training day to finish. "I don't mind waiting until tomorrow," I said, hoping I sounded flexible. *Yah, off the hook today.*

Back at my apartment, I leaned my cane against the wall and left a trail of messiness behind. I eased myself into the recliner and elevated my feet. "Mo," I said when he answered my call, "are you sitting down? You're never going to believe everything that happened to me today." Without my sleep shades, I felt normal again. "It all started with the elevator...."

Mo had met with the Office of Disabilities and, together, they hashed out some strategies for the coming term. "My first task is to get a list of the text books I need, and they'll make sure they're recorded for me."

We were both moving forward.

My days settled into a pleasant pattern. I had evaded the mobility instruction by not volunteering for three days, but couldn't put it off any longer. I had to get past my fear of the instructor watching me do something wrong.

When I finally left for my first lesson, I discovered Joe's way of teaching was different from my previous instructor. Everyone had his own style, I reminded myself. Just be flexible.

Joe seemed like a by-the-book cop. He walked fast, spoke sharply and interjected often—a bit on the gruff side.

"Put your hand this way," he ordered, rapping me on the knuckles and repositioning the fingers of my right hand on the cane.

My face grew hot. I hadn't even mastered the right way to grip a cane in all those months. *Don't be silly,* I told myself, *there might be multiple ways to grip a cane.*

From the cool breeze and smooth sidewalks, I guessed our session took place in an upscale, tree-lined neighborhood. I huffed as I climbed uphill, finding the curb with my cane. I stopped, unsure if I should go ahead and listen to the traffic or wait for Joe to tell me when to cross.

"Where are we, Joe?"

"Shaker Heights. All my clients like this area. Old homes, big bucks in Cleveland. Million dollar houses. You let me know when you feel it's safe to cross," he added.

I listened, my body rigid, as I ascertained the level of safety before crossing. Then I realized the neighborhood was not much different from the ones in the suburbs of Erie, and I crossed without difficulty.

Joe described the old Tudor houses and their landscaped yards. "Quite a few of the homes go back to the 1920s."

"Really?"

It struck me how our walk through Shaker Heights was more like a fun tour than a lesson. Even when I couldn't see, I could picture everything, even the train tracks and elementary school Joe described. I made a mental note to tell Mo. After our lesson, as we returned to the Sight Center, I wondered how Mo was familiarizing his way around campus and how his experience compared to mine. Was his liaison kindly describing his route and giving him tours?

Every day at the Sight Center presented different experiences as I learned about new innovations to help the blind. "Accessibility features" only meant, 'This is how a blind person can do the same things a sighted person can do.' It lost a little of its sting.

My companions knew a lot about audio book programs, descriptive narration for movies, talking timers and other gadgets to help in the kitchen and even computerized Braille software. It boggled my mind to hear of so many ways to help blind people lead fuller lives.

I also loved keeping up with what my companions were practicing. Mark was learning how to pour liquids. There was a little battery-like device he attached to the inside of a glass. He poured water into the glass and the device beeped when the liquid neared the top. Sometimes he missed the glass, so when it worked out, we cheered.

Luisa was flying through her Braille, typing up several recipes to take home with her. I learned she was a regional spokesperson to the American

Federation for the Blind. As part of the perks, she tested a lot of innovations and wrote reviews on them.

The five of us—counting the coordinator and assistant—got along well. We played games such as Uno and Monopoly in Braille and looked forward to the next food of the day. I made applesauce with the help of a juicer and I had little cuts on my hand to prove it after I washed the components. Sometimes our food smelled so good, people in nearby offices stopped by to test-taste it. I started to feel more confident with my companions.

Mobility was going all right too. The first lesson seemed relatively easy. I think Joe wanted to gauge my skill level. In subsequent lessons, I learned to use an eyeglass monocle to find specific addresses. In another lesson, I took the monocle to the grocery store to find unit prices and read the aisle banners. Joe gave me a list of food to shop for and actually timed how long it took to gather everything. I also learned how to pull a grocery cart so I could navigate with my cane. Outdoors, I crossed streets in downtown Cleveland and tried out different shades of sunglasses to see which worked best for me. I managed the tasks without losing face.

Until...crunch! *Uh-oh.* I slowly opened the car door.

Yes, I had closed it on my cane. The bottom third dangled drunkenly.

What was I going to do? I loved my cane! Or so I felt at that moment.

"Looks like ya' did a number on that fella." The coach I had come to like switched to his 'Officer Joe' persona as he took the cane from my hands. In the silence that followed, he must have inspected it. "Ya' done killed 'im."

That made me feel even worse. As if I had murdered my cane. Maybe if I were lucky enough, I could get the charge reduced to manslaughter. I hung my head. Mobility training was over for me. I had almost made it all the way through, but this was not the way to exit. It still mattered what Officer Joe thought.

My doleful look must have softened the old boy's heart, because he said, "Hey, these things happen." Joe chucked me on the chin. "Buck up, we'll get ya' another one. Yep, we'll getcha back out there for a final lesson."

No time in the slammer? He isn't going to book me after all? I brightened. When we arrived in the parking lot at the Sight Center, I cradled the broken part in my hands. It still hung pathetically. I couldn't bear it and quickly put it out of sight in my bag.

Joe opened the car door and helped me out of the vehicle, placing my arm firmly in the crook of his arm, and took me back to our training area. I survived an error he had seen me make. Nothing terrible happened to me. I faced it. Even though breaking my cane seemed like a little thing, getting past it made me feel brave.

That night when I told Mo about the incident, he clucked, "Ya' killed your cane? I don't know if I can continue to hang out with the likes of you. You can't meet my mom now. What would I say, 'This is Amy, the cane killer?'"

"Oh you." It seemed funny now. "If I had planned a funeral in our office, we would have had to find a minister. But get this...no one would've had to wear black. No one would ever know." I got the giggles, which set Mo off. I couldn't believe I was making jokes about what people could or couldn't see. It felt good to let go, as if I were releasing some of my pent-up fears.

When the three weeks came to an end, Shirl, my counselor from Erie, traveled to Cleveland to get input on my training from the instructors and discuss the outcomes with me. "When I first met you, Amy, you were so timid. You seem to have come into your own," she observed. "That often happens when you're immersed in training."

"Yeah. Yeahhhh." I felt elated.

That afternoon, I packed my bags and made a final call from Cleveland to Mo. But no one answered. He might have been on campus finishing up his preparations. His classes started the following week. He had a full course load.

I sat on the stool at the breakfast bar and thought about how far I had come in three weeks. That pimply, nervous teenager I felt like when I had arrived and who was so dependent on Mo for reassurance wasn't gone yet. She still popped up too frequently.

But something inside me had changed. The long interactions with Luisa, Mark, Betty, Joe and, of course, Mo, left their mark on me. I could talk about blindness without feeling my stomach clench and I had a notebook of solutions and addresses for resources tucked away in my bag.

I thought about how embarrassed I had been to say or do the wrong thing around blind people or as a blind person around sighted people. But I was adjusting myself, not only in how I responded, but also in the area of control. I didn't need to appear like I had it all together. That gave me a sense of independence.

My cell phone rang. Of course, it was Mo. Still in my philosophical mood, I said to him, "Mo, do you remember when I asked you how the view was?"

"How could I forget?" We both had a laugh. Then he said, "Okay, Grandma, I got a question for you. I been hearing about Amy's adventures every single night. You boo-hooed about your cane and almost burnt the place down cooking Japanese tempura in hot oil. I wanna know. After three weeks, what's the view like on *this* side of blindness?"

"Mo, you get an 'A' for that question! It must be all those study skills I'm helping you with." I laughed. "I don't know. My view is changing.

The landscape isn't pretty or serene, but it's not as dark or dreary as it used to be. How and what I see depends as much on my attitude and outlook as what my eyes show me."

"Hey, Grandma, now you're seeing a little bit of the same view I see in Edinboro. You're gonna have some really ugly views. But at the end of the day, remember the sun sets on your goals too. When you reach 'em, the view is gonna look beautiful and feel sweet."

6/ STAGE FLIGHT

A year before my memoir came out, I received my first invitation to speak. A friend from my college days heard I was writing a book. She had volunteered to serve on the Ladies' Retreat committee at her church and needed a speaker. She wrote in bold print, "Have you ever been a keynote speaker?"

I gulped. Quickly writing back, I wrote in capital and bold letters, "NO!" I added in smaller letters, "But I'm willing to give it a shot."

Later I wondered if I meant self-inflicted *gun*shot because when she wrote back, she said it would be fun to see me again, and if I wanted it, the job was mine. How much would I charge?

Did I want it? Should I take it?

With nothing to compare it with, I responded, leaving it up to chance. "Whatever the budget of your women's ministry allows."

Afterward, I vacillated between confidence and terror.

Sometimes when I imagined myself in this role, I danced around the apartment singing little rhymes like, "I'm the lady of the hour. So bring it on, God, anoint me with Your Power!" Other times I would lay my head on my computer desk and despair. "I'm never going to finish this book in time. I might as well resign as a speaker."

I had a wide range of fears—from the typical speaking *faux pas*, such as tripping as I walked up to the podium or blanking out in the middle of my message, to fielding questions afterward. My drastic recent drop in vision brought on a different set of fears. Some of them—especially the ones that came to me in bed—teetered on the ridiculous. What if I stood on the wrong side of the podium and addressed my talk to the back wall and no one told me until afterward? Or worst case scenario—what if my mobility cane caught on the step and, when I pulled it loose, it knocked over the podium, which would in turn rip the cable from the wall, naturally tossing my CD player into the air and making it land with a thud on the wrecked stage?

Although my mind jumped to the most alarming possibilities, I knew this was a great opportunity. A keynote speaker for someone who was just starting out in a new career! What could be better? Any time a member of my church asked about it, I pumped my arm into the air three times. "I. Can't. Wait!"

The book was progressing, but not fast enough. I had agreed to speak about my vision loss and how God worked to meet the needs of vision loss as well as other losses in my life. Afterward, I would sell my book. Isn't that what featured speakers at ladies' retreats did? That's what my writing coach said and I followed it like a prescription.

Only...I didn't finish the book in time. So I chose Esther, a courageous woman from the Bible, to put my talks into context. God used her to save a whole nation of people. I would show her journey from fear to faith since I had faced that scenario in my vision loss and in my attempts to have children.

First I had to make Esther's situation clear. Since she had to endure a year of beauty treatments in hopes of pleasing and possibly marrying the king, I looked through my photographs of the Middle East and chose three photos to tell Esther's story. I decided to blow them up and create a poster on foam board. The first and largest photo was of a glitzy princess. In the next square, I added some fancy gold bottles of perfume and incense on a mirrored tray. I finished the poster with a photo of a bride's foot and hand decorated in traditional designs using henna—a natural dye and part of any Middle Eastern wedding celebration.

Satisfied that my first-hand knowledge of the customs similar to those Esther likely faced would catch their attention, I finished my preparations. After packing a carry-on bag of devotional books to sell, which included pieces of my writing, I was ready.

That sunny afternoon in May, my driver, Judie, and I headed across the state line to Lakemount Church in New Waterford, Ohio. There I would meet my college friend and drive on to the hotel. The Ladies' Retreat started early the next morning.

We arrived and my college pal, Wendy, met me in the church foyer. "It's been thirty years and you haven't changed a bit!" she cried, giving me a once-over.

Uh....My vision had changed a little bit! I wanted to wave my cane in a figure eight to demonstrate I knew that change was why I had been selected to speak. But I didn't. I held it straight up and down. "You look great too!" I chirped and introduced her to Judie. After catching up, Wendy asked if I'd like to see where I'd be speaking.

"Uh, sure," I said, wondering if she noticed my slightly high-pitched, uncertain response. As I followed her to the sanctuary, I swept my cane back and forth.

Inside the dark room, Wendy introduced me to another committee member. I set my cane aside at a corner pew and shook her hand warmly.

"Hey, girl," Wendy pointed to a platform. "You'll be speaking up there." I followed her finger to the raised stage and walked toward it. *Urgh! Forgot my cane.* Too lazy to backtrack, I brushed the importance of my cane aside.

"This is how the schedule will work. The program will start at nine.

We have five other speakers. I will introduce each one."

I nodded several times, as I figured keynote speakers do to show how savvy they are.

"Two women from our church will speak before you do, then you go on for your session. We'll break for lunch. Afterward, you'll deliver your second session, but keep it to half an hour, forty-five minutes max, because three others will give talks after you."

"I won't go over." I hoped my talk would last long enough.

"Why don't you go up and get a feel for the stage?" she suggested.

I carefully stepped up to the podium.

"Speech. Speech," Judie called.

I cleared my throat and, imagining myself another Abraham Lincoln, said playfully, "Four score and seven years ago, I mean, in nineteen seventy-eight, I made a friend at a small college in West Virginia...." I started to walk across the stage in front of the podium as I expanded on my speech. I imagined myself another Benjamin Franklin and waxed poetic in my lighthearted mood. "Nearly thirty years after our graduation, on this auspicious day tomorrow and on this very stage...."

At that moment, I walked off the stage.

My friends gasped.

"It's all right, ladies, nothing to worry about. As you can see, I landed on my feet between the platform and the communion table. I'm a little thirsty and thought this would be the fastest way to the wine...."

As the committee members patted me down to be sure I hadn't chipped any bones, Judie deadpanned, "Amy, I thought you'd gotten over your stage flight."

Wendy and the other committee member exchanged worried glances. My ol' college pal rallied a response, "Well, if you haven't, I'm grounding you tomorrow."

"Please, Mommy, don't ground me. I'll stick to the stage."

*****

After we settled into our hotel, the church elder and his wife took us out to dinner at a fancy German restaurant in the area. *Nice restaurant, nice hotel, transportation allowance. This keynote speaker job is pretty cool.* I ate so much that evening I felt I'd have to walk several laps in the hotel hallway to fit into my clothes the next morning.

As Judie lay down to sleep, my nerves got the better of me, and I practiced my talk in the bathroom. The next morning, I slipped out of bed early, showered and dressed and continued to practice my two topics. I had a queasy feeling in the pit of my stomach that wouldn't go away. Judie tapped on the bathroom door. "How's it goin'?"

I opened the door. "Don't ask." The reflection in the mirror showed a white face. My lips were drawn in a clown-like grimace. I quickly looked away.

"You'll do fine." She leaned in. "Your earrings are on the wrong ears."

"What!"

Each earring was a delicate blue eye with a zirconium border, hanging inside a much larger silver teardrop shape. A friend from my sight support group had made them for me to celebrate my first speaking engagement. I looked in the mirror again. She was right. Only the silver backing showed. "Oh my gosh!"

"It's all right." Judie's voice was calm. "Just switch ears."

"Switch *ears?*" In my state, I imagined myself taking off one ear and putting it where the other one was. "That's a little drastic to fix my problem, don't you think?"

"No, silly. I mean, switch *earrings* from one ear to the other," she corrected. "Trust me, that'll work."

When I transferred my earrings to the opposite ears, with a bit of finagling by Judie, the blue eye faced the proper direction. After my initial relief, I started doubting my entire appearance. "Is my shirt on okay or is it inside out? Are my pants on backward? Where are my glasses? Um...."

"Your glasses are to your right. You look fine. How do you feel about your talk?"

"All I can remember is my name and how I know Wendy. I'm all jangly." I took several breaths to compose myself.

When we arrived at the church, Wendy hurried in. "Do you want to wear a headset with a mike or use a regular microphone like the rest of the women?"

Headset gear? No way. I didn't want any 'special treatment' because of my vision loss. I imagined wearing a headset with some space age mike system looped outside my brain. "I'll use what everyone else is using."

I stood next to Wendy, a frozen smile on my face, my heart thudding in my chest. How would I make it through the next half hour?

"...So, without further delay, I will turn the stage over to our keynote speaker."

I stepped up to the podium holding the microphone in my trembling fingers. When I scanned the nearly one thousand attendees, I quaked. But I could only see those in the first few rows. The rest of the audience blurred. That helped. I was in the middle of sharing an exposé of my college classmate and her daring 'pink gang' when I noticed my voice coming over the sound system in a strange pattern—megaphone loud then quiet.

"...So wearing pink T-shirts, the all-female band raided the men's dorm and stole the underwear of five especially fortunate gentlemen. They hung them onto an outdoor clothes line in front of the women's dorm...."

The "dorm" came out loud. I sounded like a giant. I tried to hold the mike still. But I moved around a lot, so I found myself leaning in and moving away from the microphone. I could hear my voice fluctuate in intensity, but I didn't know how it sounded to the listeners. Was it as loud as it seemed or was that because I used the handheld mike?

After a while, I felt like a see-saw, with my voice pumping up and down. I didn't know how to jump off safely. If I didn't speak into the microphone, no one would hear me, so I continued on and hoped for the best.

Two-thirds of the way through my talk about Esther and coping with my vision loss, when I turned over a note card, the microphone bumped the other cards and they flew off the podium. Judie stepped onto the stage and handed them to me. If people hadn't noticed the accident at first, they surely did then. I didn't need those silly note cards anyway. I should have tossed them up in the air at the start of the talk and said, "Let's just talk woman to woman, friend to friend." At least it would have got a laugh.

Finally, my session finished and we broke for lunch.

"How did I do?" I asked Wendy, breathlessly.

"Oh yeah, great." She gave me a thumbs-up, but didn't make eye contact with me. "Have to run to make sure everything goes smoothly at the luncheon." She dashed away.

I headed off to the restroom to freshen up and collect myself. When a woman from my home congregation came over to me at the sink, she hesitated then said, "Amy, I think that microphone is quite strong. You don't have to lean in to speak. It's really loud...and we can...hear you...even breathing."

I gasped, "No-o-o. Really?"

"And I don't want to hurt your feelings, but you aren't even looking at the right side of the auditorium where I'm sitting."

"Oh, goodness, you're all blurry over there. Sorry."

I wanted to run back home. I would escape to my room and throw a pillow over my head...forever. My stomach felt wretched—tight and queasy at the same time. Maybe I was too sick to finish my talk.

"Why don't you try the headset?" Judie countered, rinsing her hands and pulling a paper towel from the machine. As usual, unruffled and collected, she seemed to know my thoughts.

"We-e-l-l, I have to speak anyway. They're paying me. Yes, I will."

During the luncheon, I spoke to Wendy about the headset. "Oh yes, I'll get it for you before we start again. That will be super," she enthused.

When I gave my second talk, I walked across the stage so naturally and looked out at my audience in each of the three sections.

No stumbling. No pausing. No flying. Everything went smoothly. I shared how Esther, now the queen and facing possible death, found her courage "at such a time as this" to reveal her Jewish identity to King Mordecai and sway his decision on a death sentence to the Jews.

In this session, I gave my testimony about how I found the courage to reach out to women of many nationalities in a hospital pregnancy ward as I faced the loss of my twins. It was an emotional and yet hope-laden talk. The headset gave me added freedom and confidence. After the technician played the inspirational song on my CD—"God Use Me" by Andy Landis, an Australian singer songwriter—there wasn't a sound in the auditorium, except for sniffing and women blowing their noses. My message had reached their hearts.

At the next break, several women came up to me and shared stories of their childbearing losses and miscarriages. "And with your sight issues, I'm sure it was even more difficult," someone said.

One young woman sobbed, "That song was beautiful, exactly what I needed to hear. I still can't believe my baby…died."

It didn't require good sight to see a woman's raw pain. I held her close as her shuddering sobs slowly ebbed away. Though I had planned to focus mostly on how I thrived with ongoing vision loss, the message that touched most of the women that day was how I moved forward after losing my twin girls.

I can't help but feel God opened the door through my vision loss, but used me to begin the healing journey for mothers still mourning those little lives ripped away too soon.

In spite of the mishaps I experienced as a rookie keynote speaker, they were not cane-related. None of my far-fetched fears came to pass. When I needed to, I moved with confidence and grace. My cane not only aided me but also gave my walk and talk legitimacy. It was only several weeks later that I even realized that my earrings were identical and it was impossible to put them in the 'wrong' ear.

Something must have gone right on the stage that day, because after the women's retreat, my speaking engagements took flight. Invitations came, and when I finished my book, I was ready to meet the new demands of my career.

7/ RUNNING A FINE LINE

Even when you're going blind like me, running is a great source of exercise and enjoyment that makes it worth pursuing. As one foot after the other pounds the pavement, I feel alive and think about blisters, speed, distance and feeling fit like every other runner. More than anything, running makes me feel as if I'm still living life my way.

My running has taken many forms—from timing myself as I dashed to my friends' houses and back as a child to regularly running hills with a friend in high school. I even found a way to keep up my passion overseas by joining Hash House Harriers, an international running club. Each month, we sprinted along planned routes that took us through rice paddies, along tropical beaches and, in one country, the Arab Gulf.

Being a vision-impaired runner overseas was a great way to make international friends. I discovered this when I took a wrong turn in a chest-high rice paddy. "Help!" brought Japanese, Chinese and a German runner to my rescue.

By the time I moved back home, my vision loss had progressed to the point where running through my neighborhood endangered me. If a sewer grating didn't trip me up, then the uneven sidewalk did. After I received my cane, I experimented by trying to run with it. I should have videotaped those attempts for *America's Funniest Home Videos*. Not only did I keep outrunning my cane, I also looked like a reluctant pole vaulter who never jumped forward. Now I find it best to run in a controlled area.

Luckily, the high school track is less than a mile from home. A smooth, body-friendly track works well. A tumble there doesn't leave much of a scar. Occasionally, the track and field hurdles block my path and catch me off guard, or I cross a few lanes on a bad vision day. But it isn't crowded enough to deter me. This environment enables me to pursue my running goals. When others run alongside me, the motivation is even stronger. I feel as if I'm flying down the track.

One summer night, I decided to fit in a run. When I laced up my running shoes, I noticed a Band-Aid with one end flapping and pressed the loose side down, covering the remnant of my last running fiasco. It only took a few minutes to hit the track and get into my running groove. I wondered what adventure the evening's run would bring.

It was hot and muggy, so the sweat poured off me. As I plucked my shirt from my chest to provide more air, the words a running colleague said came back to me: "Men sweat and women glisten." Hmph! When it came to running, sweat was sweat.

The bright sun suddenly blinded me. My eyes closed involuntarily, and when they opened, they veered to the right side of the track. An organized succession of black dots appeared. *Is that Braille? Why would the school put up a Braille sign in summer? How did the coach know a legally-blind runner was using the track?*

Coming up on the curve where the Braille dots were, I tried to read them and instead crashed into a chain-link fence surrounding the track. It took a moment to realize the "Braille" was actually the visible chain links that formed part of the fence. I'd crossed six lanes to "read" the Braille, but not with my hands—this time it was with my head.

Ouch! My Band-Aid dangled off my hand again and I gently removed it before setting out to resume my run.

A few more laps around and I came up with a name for the phenomenon and defined it. Light-outs: the act of running at sunset, which causes temporary blindness, occurring on the right side of the track. At the curve, I put one foot in front of the other and attempted to run straight even when the lane marker washed in and out of view.

My thoughts drifted to another temporary blindness—a weather-related phenomenon. Area residents referred to them as "white-outs." During our blustery Pennsylvania winters when I still drove, I used to pass through pockets of pure white. In our lake-effect storms, the wind whipped the snow across the highway, wiping out the sight of everything for a few seconds.

At least running blind, I worried only about the speed of my legs and not four wheels and an engine. Besides, the left side of the track arrived soon enough and my vision returned.

Better finish up here. Soon it'll be dark. I was on my seventh lap. A glance at the sky told me I didn't have much time before it was "lights out." The darkness descended swiftly, just like when my mother used to say, "Okay, lights out now. Go to sleep." The sun set on the track almost as fast.

Speeding up, I realized I ran a fine line between light-outs and lights out. It seemed strange that both the light and the darkness blinded me. My eighth lap made two miles.

Happy to reach my goal, I found my hand towel hanging on the fence, wiped the sweat off me and quickly stretched. Because I never brought my cane to the track, I had to quick-foot it home so I wouldn't get lost, even though the road was familiar.

Heading home that night, I thought of how much my running meant to me—enough to find solutions to keep pursuing my passion. The track works well for me now, but like all the other methods I have incorporated into my life to keep it going, I'll have to switch to another lane—likely leader dogs and running guides—both of which will allow me to live life on my terms.

That's life in the track lane![1]

[1] This chapter was first published in DIALOGUE, January-February 2007. For a free sample issue of DIALOGUE or information about other publications, contact Blindskills, Inc., P.O. Box 5181, Salem, OR 97304-0181; Phone: 800-860-4224; Email: info@blindskills.com; Web site: www.blindskills.com.

8/ WHEN ONE DOOR CLOSES...

Pouring down rain. Great! What a day for a craft and furniture sale.

"Hop in!" My brother loaded the cardboard boxes in the cab and put the two wooden drawers that held my cross-stitched Palestinian pillows and my Filipino crafts in the back of his pick-up along with my whiteboard where I planned to write the prices.

His windshield wipers ran full speed as he backed out of the driveway and headed to the shop to pick up his rustic furniture.

We would sell our wares at a local church.

My brother's a good guy. He carried my boxes in and set up a table for me. I only had to wipe down my containers, unload my crafts and list my prices. Being vision-impaired has its upside.

The church had more vendors than buyers. After checking out what some of the others were selling, I returned to wait. And wait. Finally, I had a buyer. She bought a fish bracelet. Score! By lunchtime, I'd given exactly one business card out and sold a couple of the Filipino wares. The afternoon was only slightly better. A short while later, I decided to make my way over to the restroom. I grabbed my cane and set out. The dreary rain made the inside of the church look darker and blurrier than it might have been otherwise.

The restroom is on this side of the building, I'm certain.

I slowed down, tentatively slid my cane back and forth a couple of times over the polished floor and paused.

"You lookin' for somethin'? Can I help ya'?"

I smiled in the general direction of the voice. "Yes, thanks. Just trying to find the bathroom." The tip of my cane was forward and doing its job, seeking some kind of crack an inch over the floor or along the wall.

"The bathroom door's right there. Can't miss it," came the pleasant voice.

"Thanks!" I said, taking the voice literally. "I knew I'd find a door...somewhere."

I leaned over and pushed *there*. Nothing happened. I pushed again. Harder. The door didn't give way at all. Finally, I realized that I was pushing against the wall.

I giggled. "Oops. I won't get very far trying to open a brick wall."

Actually, I felt ridiculous. But I forced myself to move on as I imagined everyone staring at me.

My hands moved to the left. I groped. Finally, I felt a thin lever. The door handle. Still chuckling, I turned it and disappeared into the restroom. Inside, I took a deep breath. I must have looked like a mime artist with my hands moving over the wall like that. Only instead of wearing white make-up, I had a bright red face.

Coming back out, I had to stop. Re-orient myself. A quick question and I was off toward the vendor's circle of tables. I moved steadily across the room. When I heard my brother's voice, "Stop. You're back," I knew I'd reached my destination. I folded my cane neatly and placed it under the table.

That afternoon, with few customers to distract me, I had plenty of time to think. I learned something from taking my trek to the bathroom. First of all, it's really frustrating when someone who obviously sees you are navigating with a cane directs you to a location with a "right there." Where actually is "there?" To the right? To the left? No wonder I was having difficulty finding it for myself.

I was so ready to take all the responsibility...or the blame...for my mistake. But negotiating directions in a strange place is a dual effort. I think I have to overtly tell people, "I'm visually impaired. Can you tell me where the bathroom door is?" If they hear those words, it will remind them that I can't see "there" and need specific directions. Then I will avoid this kind of predicament.

But sitting there with my crafts, I found the humor. Remember that old adage, "When one door closes, another one opens...?" Today I can safely add, "Or maybe, one isn't even a door at all!"

9/ EXIT STAGE LEFT, CUE LAUGHTER

Thunk. Huh? I moved my long white cane sideways. *Thunk.* In the opposite direction. *Thunk.* Backward. *Thunk.* I could barely move. I stepped forward. *Bam.* My head smacked into something flat and hard. Out of habit, I reached up to feel for blood. At that moment, I knocked something else over. It sounded like a tin can. I turned around in a full circle. Seemed like terribly cramped quarters. My hand brushed something long and bristly.

I bumped into another object—a plastic bottle? I cupped my hand around something. Yes, a nozzle. I lifted it and took a whiff. Ammonia. When my foot hit something else, I maneuvered myself to discover what—something long, thin and smooth projected out of a curved base. I followed it down to the floor. It felt suspiciously like...a mop handle and bucket.

"Wait a minute. This is not where I want to go. This is a walk-in janitor's closet!"

You might think it odd I found myself bumbling around in a janitor's closet, but for me, a woman losing her vision, jams of this sort happened frequently. Normally, I don't mind. This time, I happened to be at a writers' conference. Just outside this closet stood a well-known speaker in the Christian publishing field with a very promising message. I could hear the rise and fall of his voice and people laughing on the other side of the door.

How did I wander into the closet in the first place? I had signed up to speak to a literary agent. Ongoing interviews with publishers and agents took place throughout regular speaking sessions as a perk to attendees. Writers looking to match their talents to industry needs quietly slipped in and out of the scheduled presentations to pitch their ideas and get a foot in the door.

The key word—quietly. I didn't do much quietly. Now, I had a dilemma.

I could stay put until the session ended so I wouldn't interrupt or further embarrass myself. But then I would miss the exciting appointment with the agent. What's worse, the group might pity me when they found out I stayed in the closet for an hour.

I could burst out of the closet and say, "Wrong room. The agent is not here," chuckle and exit through the other door. Or I could say, "Surprise. Avon calling!" In the worst case scenario, I could remain behind the closed door and shout, "The sound system is not very good in here. Could you please speak a little louder so I don't miss anything?" I giggled.

How could I handle this situation with dignity?

The most sensible choice would be to exit, stage left.

I gathered my courage and stepped back into the room again. The speaker halted and heads riveted toward me. They seemed to have forgotten I entered the closet minutes earlier. I directed my loveliest smile to my fellow writers and waved goodbye. "Thank you," I mouthed to the speaker, giving him a thumbs-up for his talk and exited.

I took a deep breath and made my way to the main forum. A conference organizer scuttled over. "May I help you?"

"The Seymour Agency, please."

She guided me to the table herself and announced to the agent that I had arrived for my 10:00 a.m. appointment.

I held out my hand to greet the agent. She had a brisk, firm grip. After sitting down, I launched into my elevator pitch about *Fading Light*, the memoir I dared to peddle. And which one day I promise to publish!

*****

The frequent mishaps my vision loss caused during the conference stirred up laughter and plunked me right into the lives of other aspiring writers. Friendships developed rapidly.

Standing in line for our meal that first day, I accidentally slapped the legs of the woman ahead of me with my cane. But she didn't seem angry. One thing led to another, and she asked me how long I'd been writing.

"Professionally, a couple of months. This is a career change," I declared.

"Me, too. Welcome to the club."

Side-stepping formality, I had the time of my life. We shared common hopes for our writing, putting the bounce in our words and finding encouragement in our similar walks of life—although mine would be with a cane.

The last morning, I tapped the shoulder of a woman from one of my sessions. She stood out to me because she wore hearing aids, yet had participated in a lively discussion. After we introduced ourselves, she snapped her fingers. "I know who *you* are." She giggled. "You pranced out of the closet, gave us that dazzling smile and left the room. It took us all by surprise, but we had a good laugh."

"Yep, that's me all right."

We talked a little about the challenges we faced. She mused, "Confidence has little to do with what you can see or hear. It has everything to do with how you feel about who you are."

"Yeah, it's about how you approach life," I agreed.

We shook hands and parted ways.

On the flight back to Pennsylvania, I realized that confidence started with courage. Courage to me meant being brave enough to step out from behind that door, even if it caused everyone to turn away from the speaker and stare at me walking out of a janitor's closet filled with mops, brooms and wet rags. If I wanted to have courage, I needed to reveal my dreams to others and not hide them, the way I was tempted to hide earlier.

I couldn't be afraid to step away from my comfort zone.[2]

---

[2] This chapter was first published in DIALOGUE, January-February 2007. For a free sample issue of DIALOGUE or information about other publications, contact Blindskills, Inc., P.O. Box 5181, Salem, OR 97304-0181; Phone: 800-860-4224; Email: info@blindskills.com; Web site: www.blindskills.com.

10/ IF THE COAT FITS

"Let's go and get you squared away at the hotel," my new and remarkably energetic friend, Sally, said at the end of a long conference day.

I spied my coat hanging near the door. "It's so nice of you to volunteer to take me," I said through a yawn.

"Happy to do it." She gestured in the direction of a coat rack some distance away. "Grab your coat."

I unclasped the elastic and my cane fell into place. Barging forward, I made it in short order to where the coats hung. My cane rested against the silver clothes bar while I slid my coat off the hanger. I slung it over my shoulder, too lethargic to even put it on.

Sally courteously stepped ahead of me to get the door.

"Brrr," I said, stepping into the Kansas wind.

"You'd better wear your coat," my friend advised. "The wind has kicked up a notch since this afternoon. I don't know what it's like in Pennsylvania, but Kansas in November is pretty harsh."

"Huh?" I strained to hear her through the rattling wind. "Oh-h. My coat. I'll be fine." And continued on my way, my coat in hand.

As always, it took my eyes time to adapt to the darkness. My night blindness made it difficult to see anything. I relied heavily on her voice to guide my fumbling steps as I caught glimpses of the shadowy figure I hoped was Sally. I sped up and in doing so, lost her.

"*Sallleee,*" I called as I peered into the darkness around me. This happened to me all the time at night. People simply disappeared. Luckily, it was usually my eyes fooling me, so I never became too worked up. But in an unknown location and on a cold night like tonight, it spooked me. I imagined how easy it would be for me to blow off onto the Kansas prairie like some hapless tumbleweed, and redoubled my efforts to keep track of my friend.

"Over here, Amy!"

Sally backtracked to where I'd veered off. I held onto the cuff of her coat and let my cane skip behind me like a wandering child dawdling at its own pace.

When we arrived at Sally's car, she aimed her key at the passenger door and with a click of a button, unlocked it. "It's open," she said and dashed around to the driver's side.

I uncurled my fingers, still wrapped around the black handle of my cane, and leaned my stick against the door frame. The cane promptly fell. I addressed it, "Okay, be that way. You'll just have to wait." I opened the back door and dropped my coat onto the seat. Tossing my briefcase into the dark carpeting, my purse fell on top of it. With my hands finally free, I reached over and picked up my cane. "In you go," I said as I folded it up and placed it on the floor.

Sally blew on her fingers. "Hop in!"

A sudden gust of wind tossed me into the vehicle. "The wind moves at the sound of her voice!" I grinned and folded up my cane. "H-h-eat, p-please!"

"Coming right up." She turned the key in the ignition and slid the lever to the maximum heat setting. "Time to get this baby rolling."

The heater defrosted the windshield, and soon we were on our way. When we arrived, Sally watched me gather all my gear together. "Why don't you put on your coat?" She suggested. "You'll have less to carry."

"That's okay, I'm used to juggling lots of things wherever I go. Thanks so much for the ride. See you tomorrow."

The next morning, I woke up early and got ready for the conference. Then I decided to go down to the lobby and get some orange juice and a doughnut.

I gathered up that day's schedule and shrugged into my coat. When I stepped over to the dresser to pick up my purse, I nearly tripped. What...? My eyes traveled down to the hem. The coat hung to my ankles.

I frowned as I dug through one pocket, feeling for my lipstick. No tube of Coral Me Crazy to be found, but my fingers grabbed onto a crumpled tissue and...one glove. I checked the other pocket. No glove there. "Hey, this is weird." *Did I drop one or something? Did I even bring my gloves to Kansas? If I did, I didn't wear them last night.*

I ran my hand down the length of the coat and felt a smooth, diamond-thread design sewn into the cloth. *It must be inside out,* I thought, wondering how I could forget that the coat was reversible. I stuck one arm through the sleeve and reversed it, then the other.

Something still didn't look right.

In a moment of playfulness, I flipped my big hood up; the tip came to my nose!

What was going on?

I ducked over to the mirror. A dwarf looked back at me. Not only that, but my coat was inside out.

"Wait a minute. My hood has fake fur around it!" This had none. I squinted to see better and inspected the light gray color that engulfed me. "Hey, my coat is darker. Purple." I slid my hand over the material. "Nylon." Mine was suede leather. This looked *nothing* like my coat except for the big hood. Wrong color. Wrong size. Wrong design.

I covered my mouth and giggled into my hands. And, ta-dah! Wrong owner!

I couldn't believe I made such a mistake. How on earth had it happened?

When Sally picked me up, I told her my dilemma. She said, as if it were the most natural mistake in the world and happened every day, "Well, put it back. The owner will claim it soon enough."

At the conference center, I furtively looked around before sliding my cane forward and over to the coat rack. Ever so casually, I hung up the imposter coat then sped away. With a cup of coffee in hand, I spied on the rack for a few minutes to see if anyone came to claim the "stolen" coat. But then the conference began and I abandoned my espionage operation. I laughed at myself trying to spy when so much of what I saw was a blur.

That evening, I selected my coat with care, double-checking for the suede leather and my fake fur white trim around the hood. The length was right. It was the correct color. The ultimate test, the pockets. If I had any doubts, they fled when my fingers found only the Coral Me Crazy tube of lipstick in my right-hand pocket—and no gloves.

Back in the hotel room, I changed into my flannel pajamas and sipped a glass of tap water. When I reached over to charge my nearly-dead cell phone, it rang immediately. It was my friend, Julio, calling to see how the day had gone.

"You'll never believe what happened—"

"I always expect to hear the worst," Julio interrupted. "What happened *this* time?"

"I'm so glad I amuse you," I said, but began to tell him the strange story.

He interrupted me, "You always add irrelevant details. Just get to the point."

When I finished telling him what happened, there was a long silence. "Say something!"

"I'm rolling my eyes. Didn't it occur to you to…actually *wear* it? At least you would've known right then you made a mistake and could've put it back."

"Well, I was too…pooped to put it on."

"Is that your attempt at alliteration?" he said and continued on his typical banter. "So because you were too 'tired,' some poor, exhausted soul arrived at the coat rack expecting to find her long, warm winter coat—which she definitely would have worn as any sane person would have done in November—had it been there. But not having it, you forced her to trek out to her own car in sub-zero Kansas temperatures. She was likely parked at the farthest end of the parking lot."

"Oh, be quiet!" I laughed, wiggling the phone charger cord in my hand to hear better. "It wasn't *that* cold."

"What possessed you to take a coat that didn't resemble your coat in any way?"

"Maybe my cane possessed me."

"That's right, blame the one tool that is most helpful to you in getting around."

I thought about it. "Well, it was an RP moment, I guess."

"What, pray tell, is an RP moment?"

I loved talking to Julio, even when he used that tone of voice. It beat coming back to an empty hotel room and obsessing about the mishaps that happened away from home. Talking to Julio put them in perspective.

"An RP moment is exactly like a senior moment, except it involves tricks my eyes are playing on me," I informed him loftily as I made it up. "It's unexplainable and always embarrassing. It's like when I mistake a fence post for a person and wave. Or dump the cooked pasta into the wrong side of a strainer. It's like when I mean to put a bunch of files on the counter. Except they miss it and scatter all over the floor with the papers spilling out everywhere. It's like—"

"I get it already. All right. I gotta go now. You better get to bed so you can wake up on time for the last day at the conference. It's another day…and I'm sure more memorable incidents."

"Thanks for the vote of confidence."

"Ha! Get some sleep."

I never knew why I picked up such a different coat. Did I see mine and reach for the one next to it? Was I that tired? Why didn't I put it on?

Just call me crazy, but sometimes it seems to me that God feels I need a good laugh to revive me and He uses my low vision to supply me with RP moments to do just that.

My take-away from this winter coat fiasco was: make sure the coat fits…first!

11/ I DIDN'T SEE THE FLOOD

The advertising jingle for Mounds Almond Joy candy bars often plays its tune in a repetitive cycle in my head. Sometimes I actually do feel like a nut. Not an almond, or a Brazil nut or even a coconut, just a nutty person. And it's all because of my unpredictable poor vision. With my RP, I get myself into strange predicaments, either because I only see part of what is happening or I don't see it at all. To make it worse, I don't know what I'm *not* seeing. These incidents often cause unexpected...shall I say, diversions, which keep me and those around me entertained.

After a big church gathering one day, that sweet southern hospitality kicked in, and I was invited to stay on for a potluck meal. In line, a friendly, somewhat older gal struck up a conversation with me, and the fellow in a western bow tie and cowboy hat in front of me turned around and joined in. I marveled at the warmth of such strangers.

The red-headed lady and I loaded up our plates and found some empty seats. Carlie, as she was called, set down her plate and pointed to the part of the room where the beverages sat. "There's a table with drinks over there. Can I help you get something?"

This cane of mine is quite the thing to get me out of my shell—and out of work. I smiled. "No, I'll be fine thanks. I'm not thirsty yet."

A little while later, I changed my mind. The thought of a glass of sweet iced tea seemed to fit the bill. "I'll be right back," I whispered, making my way over to the refreshment table. There, I picked up the only cup, a Styrofoam one, and placed it under the nozzle of the large iced tea container and flipped the lever forward.

Whoosh! The cup flew to the floor.

Uh-oh. I bent over to pick it up, but forgot that the iced tea was still flowing out since I didn't actually see it. Suddenly, I heard it. To hide what I thought was a little mistake, I thrust the cup under the spigot again to catch the iced tea.

A woman I didn't know rushed over. "Dear, cain't you see...." That's when she spied my cane. "I mean, you cain't see it. But there's a ho-wel in the bottom of youh cup," she said, drawing out the word 'hole' as only a southerner can. "Don't worry, honey, it's...it's... allll right," the lady said, her voice sounding more than a bit panicked.

The next moment, a cascade of sweet tea shot through the cup in my hand, sending it flying once more, while the rest of the tea gushed with the unchecked power of Niagara Falls over the edge of the table.

"Turn it off, turn it off," shouted another church-going lady, speeding to the scene.

The click of high heels followed as another called, "Get that cup!" Like it was a runaway fugitive. Stop! Don't let the baddie get away.

Soon, several blurry bodies sped over to organize a lined flood patrol, passing down paper towels. With dropped jaws, they spoke in hushed words of disbelief.

"It's the strangest thing...."

"I've never seen anything like it!"

"...a ho-wel in the cup." At this point, several heads moved in to inspect the defective cup, now in custody.

I felt my face heat up several degrees as I slunk away from the small crowd. One older lady took charge and sat me down, "Now, honey, you don't worry none about this. You have youhself a slice of pe-can pie."

I picked up a fork and took a bite of my freshly-baked southern pecan pie, taking the woman's advice to heart, determined to enjoy the rest of my meal. I could hear the women, still in a state of heightened emotion, as they clustered around me once again.

The humor of it snuck in. That day I do believe I caused a flood of monumental proportions at the church social. But as an out-of-town guest—and being the owner of a long white cane—somehow got me off the hook. I liked that. And I sure loved that pecan pie.

The first lady sat down again. "Psssshhhhh," she said and covered her mouth to hide the laughter. At first, I didn't understand. Was she hushing the women? Carlie turned to me and mimicked the woman. "Psssshhhhh." She, too, dissolved in laughter. That's when I realized that they might, just might, have been imitating the sound of the escaping sweet tea! Her droll throwback set off the other woman and pretty soon everyone was laughing.

I felt like a celebrity when they started patting my back and saying, "A ho-wel in the cup!" again and again, letting their laughter flow.

Just like the iced tea.

12/ THE TROUBLE WITH TRELLISES

"Where's that spade?" I mumbled to myself, leaving the garage door open to allow more light to filter in. "I know it's hanging on the wall." I took a few hesitant steps to the right and, out of habit, reached to feel for the wooden shelf. *That garden tool shouldn't be far.* I combed the wall with my eyes. Blur. Blur. Blur. I closed my left eye and tilted my head to see better. "Abracadabra!" I said, flinging my fingers out. When I opened my eyes, a narrow black object came into view. *Ha!* That's how my eyes worked sometimes. Just like magic.

"Yoo-hoo! Amy? I'm at the door to the garage. I just got home from work."

It was my neighbor, Debbie, the flower expert. I'd called her over to help me.

"Over here." I waved at Debbie, then lifted the object off the wall, tracing the curved sides with my fingertips. My garden spade. By then, my eyes had adjusted to the dim garage. "I bought some clematis for Mom and needed help planting them."

"You're going to need more than a spade for clematis. Hate to break it to ya', but that kind of flower needs a trellis to grow properly. Tell ya' what, get the trellis, and I'll help ya' tomorrow."

"I hate to admit it, but I don't know what a trellis is."

"It's a framework for climbing plants, like roses, honeysuckle, your clematis here. Some of 'em have a lattice design. I'm sure you've seen 'em in the yards around town. You can find 'em at Lowe's or K-mart."

Not my favorite kind of store, but it was do-able.

The next afternoon, I cornered my brother outside. "Come on, Mike. We gotta go to Lowe's. Deb will be here at four o'clock, and I need to have a trellis."

He looked at his watch. "Why do you always wait until the last minute? You got money for gas?"

"'Course I do." I took out a five-dollar bill and placed it in his outstretched palm. "You know Buddy's dying to go for a ride. Can we take him?"

"I don't care, but make sure you take a sheet and don't forget his leash."

My brother was a softie like me when it came to my black Lab. Buddy was already waiting at the door and squeezed past me. He raced down the familiar path to the parked car and jumped into the back seat, excited. He seemed to think that a trellis meant "treat" in dog-speak.

When we arrived at Lowe's, my brother frowned. "If we want to make it home before four, I'd better get the gas while you get the trellis. That'll save some time."

"You're not going with me?"

"You don't want to keep Debbie waiting, do you?" He looked concerned. "Can you find it yourself?"

I tossed my head. "Of course I can." I slid the passenger door open and reached for my white mobility cane. I patted the seat. Bent down to the floor. *I forgot it!*

"What are ya' lookin' for? Your purse is right there." He pointed to my shoulder.

"Ha ha! This time it's not my purse. I forgot my cane."

"You'll be okay," my brother reassured me. "Go to the help desk and ask where the trellises are," he suggested as I stepped into the parking lot.

One thing I like about my family and have always asked of them, is that they treat me like anyone else and don't help me unless I beg them—and I wasn't anywhere near that point. I liked that they believed I could do things on my own. That gave me more confidence and allowed me to remain independent.

As Mike drove away, I squared my shoulders. Lowe's garden center loomed ahead of me. Without my cane, I faced a million potential hazards. *No choice now. Another day, another dare.*

Where to start? I found the clerk. He seemed seven-feet tall with long, long legs.

"Sure, follow me," he replied when I asked him for help.

I half-skipped and half-ran to keep up with him. He didn't even turn around. So, I had to keep right on his trail. I felt like a sparrow trying to follow an ostrich.

I hadn't gone more than five hundred feet when "Ker-plat!" I torpedoed over something wide and flat—right around knee level. When I landed, my face hit the corner of whatever it was and my knees sprawled at odd angles. After a shocked gasp, I went into automatic take-stock mode. I patted myself down. Some under-eye tenderness. No broken bones. No blood. Now if I could only get up off the floor. What did I trip over?

A red wagon filled with gardening supplies in the middle of the aisle. I could hear my mobility instructor's words in my head: *Your cane would have caught it before it caught you.*

The ostrich turned around at the crash. "Oh, my *God!* Are you okay?"

"Yes, of course." My face heated up.

He waited to see if I needed help, but I scrambled up on my own. Years of practice made me quick. "It's usually about now that people ask me if I had a nice trip." No one ever said this, but I wanted to make him smile.

"Does thi... er...happen...to you a lot?"

"Actually, yes." I smiled. "Now the trellises are...."

"This way." He resumed the lead. A few minutes later, we arrived. "Here you are. Do you need anything else?"

"No thanks, I'm good." I stood in the aisle wondering exactly where the trellises were. A step to the right brought me to...I reached out a hand. *Yes! Lawn furniture.* I crossed the aisle and leaned in, my nose nearly touching the clay pots on the shelf. They had metal linked chains attached. *Hanging baskets.* A few more steps. *Different sized pots.*

No, it's not here.

I shook my head several times. I tried my old trick. "Abracadabra!" When I opened my eyes, I saw a tall, wooden-like structure leaning against the wall. *Yeah, the trellises!* I knew it was good luck and not magic, but it felt good all the same.

Debbie said to buy white. Here's a white one. I reached out. *Stuck. Just my luck.* As I wiggled it free and pulled it out, three brown trellises crashed down on me and knocked me to the floor.

"Aaaghhh!" I peeked out through some of the openings, trying to get my breath.

An older lady came around the corner. "Are you okay?"

"Yeah," I gulped from the bottom of the pile.

"Do you need any help?"

"No-o. I'll be fine," I said, feeling anything but fine.

I'll have to work my way out of this one.

"If you're sure...." With a few looks my way—I assumed she was feeling guilty for leaving me in this predicament—she backed away.

I felt for the top trellis and shifted it off me, giving me a little more wiggle room. The next one freed me a little more. "Ugh," I grunted, after trying to hold onto all three in my right hand. They didn't weigh much, but they were awkward and wide. "Yes, got it!" The white trellis clattered to the floor as I emerged out from under it. I stood up and leaned the others against the wall.

With my arms finally free, I waved them up and down like a bird flapping its wings to make sure they still worked. Both arms skinned up and a sore elbow. Bruised knees from my earlier fall. A throbbing eye. Nothing to do but get on with it.

I turned my attention to the trellises. Where was that white one? I picked it up from where it lay on the floor and looked around for another.

Might as well get two. Dad's rule of thumb: one can never stock too many of anything. There will always be an extra one when you need it.

With the trellises in my arms, I headed for the exit. Which way was out? Everything looked the same. I had forgotten to leave bread crumbs behind me to find my way home.

First, I carried the trellises over my head, then to one side. Then to the other. I stretched to try to relieve the strain. I hated those trellises.

Careful there. Don't run into anything. Or clobber anyone. Knocking off someone's head definitely wouldn't be smart.

I tiptoed through the main aisle, trying to balance the load of trellises. Thinking of tiptoeing reminded me of an old song I hadn't thought of in years. I quietly sang to myself, "Tiptoe though the tulips with my trellises. Don't break the window...." My voice trailed away as another customer looked my way. I never could carry a tune. *Okay, time to get serious! Where's the checkout?*

I tried another direction. Dead end. How many walls *were* there here? My brother would be wondering what happened to me. What time was it? A glance at my wrist told me I'd forgotten my watch. *No watch. No cane. On a roll here.*

Finally, I saw what looked like a blue vest. "Please tell me where the exit is."

He stared at me. I saw him point straight ahead as if in slow motion. His eyes shuttered closed like two windows when he turned to me again. "Straight ahead," he said.

Whoops! Yes, it was. Less than two feet away. I reminded myself my cane would have explained why I couldn't see something so close. It wouldn't make sense to say, "I don't have my cane today, so I have to use your eyes." I was almost afraid he'd grab the trellises from my arms and stalk me. Come to think of it, except for the image of him lumbering after me, I would have welcomed him taking the horrible trellises off my hands. But he didn't. He just walked away without lifting a finger. *At least I'm safe!*

I came across the outdoor checkout. There, I saw a big guy with auburn hair. *Yah, my brother!*

He reached over and relieved me of the trellises. "Where have you been?"

"Thank you!" Boy, was I glad to hand over those trellises! "You don't want to know. Hey, can you do me a favor? I need some dirt, pleeease?"

"Do you need to get it today, or can it wait?"

"I really need it today. I want to plant Mom's clematis. That's why Debbie's coming over."

Mike was already looking around for the dirt. "All right. But this was supposed to be a quick trip," he reminded.

I chuckled. "It was a trip all right."

A few minutes later, I saw a figure. It couldn't have been my brother. The form staggered through the aisle, well, like a drunken bag of Miracle-Gro on a weekend binge. In a clever display of ventriloquism, the bag spoke. "Here I am."

A head peeked out from a life-sized bag of soil. When the bag tumbled onto the surface near the register, the rest of my brother popped out. He mopped his face with a hanky. "That's the only size I could find."

"No way! Really?"

The cashier rang everything up. "That will be thirty-five fifty," she informed me.

Uh-oh. Not enough. Despite my dad's rule of thumb, I'd have to put one trellis back. "Sorry, one is enough." I pointed to the top one on the counter.

The clerk set the other aside without comment and advised, "If I were you, I'd use a wagon to move that soil."

My brother was all for that.

In the parking lot by the car, we both stared at the bag of soil. Mike said, "You get on one end, and I'll pick up the other."

I couldn't lift my end.

"See if you can find someone to help me lift it."

Bossy. Brothers are like that. I hurried into the store. When I looked around, who did I see? My good friend, the clerk I'd dubbed Big Bird. I scurried over to him and explained about the large bag of dirt. Of course he agreed to help. This time I led. Thank goodness, there were no wagons en route to our vehicle. We parked in the handicapped section, so we didn't have far to walk. By the time we arrived, my brother had already managed to get the soil into the back seat.

"Sorry," I said. "I guess it's done."

"No problem." Big Bird waved and set off for the store.

I went around to the other side of the car to check on my dog. Buddy was squeezed into a small space a few inches from the window. He looked miserable. *Oh, Buddy.* I missed his joyful bark.

"Let's go," I said to my brother, "We'd better get Buddy home."

"Wait. Aren't you forgetting one little detail? We need to take your trellis," my brother reminded.

"Oh yeah, that's right." *How could I forget about the trellis? After all, that's why we came.*

Obviously, it didn't fit inside the car. I looked at my brother, and he looked at me. "String!" we said together.

"Go catch up with that guy," he urged. "I'll get the trellis out of this parking space and see if I can get it on the roof."

"I'll try," I said, moving as fast as I safely could. The clerk had vanished by the time I made it to the front doors of the store. Inside Lowe's, I wandered around for a few minutes. Suddenly, I collided with someone. "Sorry," I said, before realizing I had actually bumped into a pole.

Still smiling about the pole, I spotted my good pal, Big Bird. "You were waiting for me to come back, weren't you?"

"Huh? Not you again." At least I got a grin out of him. "What do you need now?"

He's enjoying this!

"String. Twine. Anything to tie that trellis down."

"Oh. I suppose you need me to help you?" he pretended like I was imposing on him.

"Nah, we'll be fine. But thanks anyway."

"Oh, come on, you need me. Really."

Was I crazy turning down his help? With the twine in hand, I set out to find my brother's car in the parking lot again.

This buying-a-trellis-job was exhausting.

Once we got the trellis tied down, my brother handed me the twine. I set it down in the parking lot.

"You can't leave it here," he protested. "Lemme take it back." He bent over, picked it up off the asphalt and walked it back to the store.

On the way home, my brother asked, "What happened to your eye? It's black."

"I dunno. I tripped over a wagon, got buried under some trellises, ran into a cement pole...the usual." *Geez! I have a black eye now! Hey, what if it's a shiner? I never had one of those before.* I peeked into the rearview mirror and craned my neck, but couldn't see my eye from any angle.

As we pulled into the driveway, I opened the door for Buddy to jump down. He stayed put. *Maybe now he thinks that 'trellis' means a bag of dirt that takes up all his space.* I realized that it was blocking the door he usually left the car from. *This might take a biscuit.*

My brother loosened the twine and lifted the trellis down from the luggage rack. He leaned it against the garage door. "You're on your own with Buddy," he said, forgetting about the dirt. I was about to remind him, but decided to tackle it myself.

I tugged at the bag of soil, both arms around it, and dragged it out of the vehicle, ripping holes and trailing dirt to the corner of the garage. I ran to get a treat for my dog. "Come on, Buddy! Look what I have for you."

Buddy picked up his head, studied the biscuit as it wiggled between my fingers. He jumped down and gobbled it up, tail wagging. He nuzzled me and smiled his toothy grin. My heart melted for just a moment as I pulled him close.

Right then, Debbie pulled into the driveway. *Four o'clock already?* "I see you got your trellis. Let's go find where to put it."

"Hang on. Let me get my cane."

I picked it up from inside my back door and followed her around the yard. As I bumped my cane over the grass in a token use of it, she turned a measured eye to the corners of my yard in her expert way.

She wasn't happy with it at first and wandered over to the side. "I found the perfect place for your trellis," Debbie finally announced. She bent over to push the stakes into the dirt, then started fiddling with something at the bottom of my trellis and looked over at me. "Amy, you can't use this one," she finally said. "It's damaged. See? It's missing two spikes. You'll have to take it back and exchange it."

"You've got to be kidding!"

She pointed to the bottom left-hand side. "Look at it."

Yes, it was broken. I didn't follow Dad's rule of thumb either. *Aagh!* I could almost feel steam coming out of my ears by that point. "This trellis is jinxed. Trellises in general are overrated. The trouble with trellises...."

If only I could blink my eyes, say "Abracadabra," and have a trellis magically appear like other objects that suddenly, out of the blue, showed up in my line of vision.

This was one instance that wasn't going to happen.

13/ IF ONLY MR. MAGOO HAD A CANE LIKE MINE

Being partially sighted for some time, I felt stressed in public because I never knew what kind of situation I would find myself in. For example, when walking my dog in the park, I often thought fence posts were people. And to me, it looked as if the low dark bushes were their dogs. It wasn't until I came near them that they reverted into fence posts again.

In malls, I sometimes reached out to touch the fabric of an outfit, only to discover that a real person was wearing it. In banks, I tried to walk through ropes.

Before I received my cane, these blunders happened frequently and, of course, without warning. Once I started using a cane, I thought all the mishaps would stop.

On one occasion, as I was walking home from the bank, I took a familiar route through town. Because I knew the way, it didn't seem like a big deal to leave my cane at home. When I reached the public library, some patrons walked out the door carrying books. My home computer was down, and I needed to check my email. I hurried in, handed the librarian my card and asked, "Just sign in for the computer?"

She nodded and resumed her work at the desk.

Along the table were four computers. The farthest from me was available, so I picked up the clipboard sign-in sheet and neatly wrote my name and time on the first line.

Before I could log on to the computer, the librarian came over and whispered something in my ear. Whatever she said was lost because I had forgotten to wear my hearing aids. But the third time, when she raised her voice a little, I finally understood. "There are some more computers around the corner. Would you like to use one of those?" she asked politely.

"Oh no, thanks, this one will be fine." The idea of wasting any more time didn't appeal to me. I hadn't checked my email in a couple of days and was waiting for a response from a publication.

The librarian stood behind me for a minute without saying anything, making me uncomfortable. I tried to ignore her. Finally, she tapped me on the shoulder and cleared her throat. "Umm, well, uh, that's not...a computer," she said with a funny look.

Much to my horror, I realized that the computer I wanted to use was actually a *picture* of a computer hanging on the wall. In fact, I then noticed the word, 'COMPUTER,' written across the top of the paper in large black font. Another instance of my shifting vision—gaps where words existed, but didn't appear until later.

Great Scot! Will I ever be able to show my face in this library again? Or even to a picture of a library?

Picking up my purse, I mustered some enthusiasm in the hope the librarian would at least find me agreeable. "In that case, I would be delighted to use the other computer. Can you show me the way?"

She turned the corner, gesturing to a single computer on the table.

I laughed—a silly titter—and said, "This will do fine."

Twenty minutes later, the librarian returned and tapped me on the shoulder. Again, a whisper that required deciphering. I caught some of the words, "...library clothes something-something blog noon."

She waited politely for some kind of response.

Feeling like a contestant on *Wheel of Fortune* with the clock ticking, adrenalin coursed through me. I paused and studied the board in my head, tossing out and rearranging letters. *Is there an 'S'?* I turned to the imaginary host. *I'm ready to solve the puzzle now, Pat.* "The library is closing, so you—rather, *I*—have to log off soon, right?"

Vanna White—I mean, the librarian—gestured her approval and glided off as the letters dinged into place.

Holding back a smile, I exited from Verizon and out of the computer altogether. The clipboard caught my eye. Should I sign out when I forgot to sign in? That *was* the rule, so I did both at the same time.

The lights in the room dimmed momentarily. The five-minute warning.

Scrambling out of my seat, I pushed the chair in and left.

When I reached the librarian's desk, the need to explain about what happened earlier came over me. "Sorry, you know, I can see—but I can't. Well, I usually have a cane. I mean, like a blind one, not one for old people—the elderly. Well, not really blind, more vision-impaired...." I grimaced. Obviously, anyone who mistakes a sign on the wall for a computer is really blind—in a Mr. Magoo kind of way.

The librarian looked more confused than ever by my explanation as I waved goodbye and backed out of the building.

The poor woman saw me enter and sign in without any problem. It looked like I had normal vision like everyone else. Partial sight is confusing that way. It betrays me when I least expect it to, so I have to be prepared with proof that my vision isn't what it appears to be. Having my cane with me would have explained why a picture of a computer looked like the real thing. I wouldn't have had to say a word. Trying to clarify low vision to others can often lead to complicated explanations.

They say a picture is worth a thousand words. I guess it depends on the picture and where it is placed. It seems a mobility cane will head off a thousand words far more easily than a picture can display even one. My cane is a valuable asset. In my world of shifting vision, I find it more and more necessary to carry my cane and let it speak for me.

14/ I'M NO SQUIGGLE

"I guess this packet of nails will work in my kitchen."

My friend, Judie, agreed. "We can always return the nails if they don't." She smothered a yawn. "Is that it, then?"

At my nod, we left for the checkout. As we passed various sets of screwdrivers, I was tempted to stop and look them over. But we had been running errands all day, and the thought of going home looked pretty good. I kept going and withdrew some bills while in line, but discovered I didn't have enough cash. This would have to go on my credit card. We reached the cashier, who rang up my purchase.

I handed him my card and waited. "Where do I sign?" I asked, looking across the counter for a receipt.

The thin, middle-aged man wearing glasses looked bored. "In the little gray box. See? There's a line?"

Oh, one of those machines. "Okay. I don't use my credit card too often, so I'm not familiar with these machines."

Unfortunately, everything looked gray in the little box. I couldn't see any line. I set my cane against the counter and leaned in to look more closely, using a scanning technique I had learned in order to bring things outside my vision into my line of sight. *Okay, there it is!* My eyes adjusted to the dark-colored box, and I picked up the attached gray instrument.

"It's really not necessary for you to sign," the man muttered, hastily taking the graphic pen from my fingers. "A squiggly line like this will do." He dashed off a line in the space. "That's fine."

What? My already creased brow wrinkled a little bit more. The cashier didn't even make eye contact with me. I bit my lip. I brought my hands together and tapped my lips before releasing them. My jaw dropped. Was it even *legal* for a stranger to sign my credit card instead of me? I was liable for that money being taken out of my account. He took the power out of my hands when he took the graphic pen away. It upset me that he took matters into his own hands.

Perhaps when he had seen the cane leaning against the counter and the fact I had asked him where to sign, he jumped to the conclusion that I was *totally* blind. Why didn't he ask me? Maybe he was trying to be helpful in his own way. He didn't want to embarrass me, so he sped things along. He probably didn't want to draw any more attention to the fact I couldn't see. I guess he thought he was being efficient in keeping the line moving.

What should I have done? I knew what my signature looked like and I just needed a little time for someone to show me where to sign. After all, my signature was part of my *identity*. Something that could never be taken from me. Even if I lost more vision, I would *still* recognize my signature. If I went completely blind, there are square cut-outs designed to help position a person's signature on a straight line. I didn't want a wavy, back-and-forth line a child could have drawn to represent me. I was quite capable on my own. I had to wonder, did this happen to other vision-impaired people?

I would have loved a moment to have had the opportunity to train the cashier to let him know I could see. But it was hardly the time for a lesson. I'm sure he wouldn't have wanted me to hold the queue up any more than necessary.

When we reached the car in the parking lot, I blew up. "That guy thought I was totally blind! Did you see what happened?"

Judie touched my shoulder and said softly, "You handled it fine. He was trying to be kind."

I crossed my arms and pouted. "Well, I'm no squiggle."

"It's just one of those days. Let it go."

Let it go? Not on my life!

We rode in silence as I mulled over my rebellious words. *I'm no squiggle.* I twisted and turned and prodded them like a scientist conducting an experiment. Finally, I spoke. "You know, Judie, way back in the late eighties when I taught English to the international military housed in Texas, I had a funny way of walking. I bent over like I was bracing myself against a fierce wind, probably to see the ground better. Teachers and students thought I was in a hurry when I moved. Some students said, 'Miss Amy, why you always rush?' It was my way of not tripping."

Judie looked like she was trying to figure out if this story had a specific purpose or if I was just reminiscing.

"And before receiving orientation and mobility training, I used to feel my way around like a big white zombie—my hands straight out in front of me." I tried to re-enact it—holding my arms out and stomping my feet—in the car seat. "Thump! Thump! Thump!"

Judie laughed at my antics.

"I don't know if I physically looked like a squiggle back then, but maybe I unconsciously felt like one, always contorting myself in different ways to see better. Now, I stand straight and tall and confident. I know my cane will find the obstacles."

"You do so well," Judie agreed.

"I'm no squiggle." I threw out my arms joyously. "I. Am. No. Squiggle."

That day I learned how a not-so-great experience brought me to a greater understanding of the person I had become: confident, secure in my use of the cane and certainly able to take care of myself and sign on any dotted line.

15/ TURNING IN CLAIMS

At sixteen, I was as excited as any of my peers when I received my driver's permit. The next school term, which started in January, I took Driver's Training. Who knew I would attempt to plough through a snow drift and get the student car stuck?

"When there's a drift that big, you're supposed to use the passing lane," huffed Mr. Stephenson, the new-driver's training instructor. He threw me a look of disbelief as he opened the door to see how well I had ploughed the car into the snow.

"Sorry, I didn't know that," I said feebly, wishing I could be buried in the snowbank instead of so stuck.

It seemed Mr. Stephenson wasn't used to rookie drivers.

That summer, my dad supervised me while I practiced driving. One afternoon in August, a fast car startled me, making my foot hit the gas pedal. I swerved, and a whirling cloud of dust bellowed above the dirt road, just before I took out the mail box. On hearing the thud, I did a double take and slammed on the brakes.

My father jumped out to inspect my dangling side mirror and the mailbox at the end of the flattened steel post. "Well, that's one way to make sure the family doesn't get the school tax bill," he said with a smile.

It wasn't until much later that I understood his comment, remembering it was time for people in my area to pay their school taxes. I couldn't believe my dad was so nonchalant about my first accident. If I was as quick in the car as he was with his dry humor, I would never worry about another accident.

We turned the claim into my parents' insurance.

Later, I heard Dad retell that story with a hint of laughter as he shook his head and finished up, "...and before I knew it, the mailbox was gone."

"It was only one," I protested.

He looked over his pipe and said, "One's enough."

But apparently, I was just getting started.

As a senior in high school, I sideswiped the family car of my classmate while I backed out of their driveway. When I jumped out and inspected both vehicles for damage, I thought everything looked fine and I had miraculously escaped with only my pride nicked.

When our phone rang later that day, I found out neither vehicle was "fine." The caller was my classmate's father, his voice tight and clipped.

"Did you by chance hit my car when you left?"

"Um, I'm not sure. Who is this?" I said, politely.

"That's hit and run! I'll need the number to your insurance company, young lady."

We turned the claim into my parent's insurance.

Other mishaps followed. My mother recalls the time when I backed into a red car when I left the old Buyers Fair, a favorite hometown department store, which sold everything from birdbaths to toddlers' dresses.

"I don't even remember that one," I said, shuddering at how many close encounters there had been over the years.

"It was bad enough for the red paint to end up on the car you drove," she said, drily. "A fender bender, if I recall. We turned a claim into our insurance."

After graduating from college, I moved back home. I didn't dare have a car while doing my studies. Finally needing my own transport, my sister sold me her old Ford Torino, which reminded me of a big green boat. I had to sit on a pillow as I sailed through traffic.

The preacher's wife, Mary Ann, and I carpooled together since we both worked in downtown Erie. Our morning commutes went well, for the most part. On the days I took the wheel, the drive was a little more...unpredictable. My nails, bitten to the quick, were proof of the near misses we drove through during rush hour traffic.

Late one afternoon, while driving home from work, Mary Ann and I were deep in discussion. We were approaching the traffic light just before the intersection on West Twelfth and Cherry when I realized I was in the wrong turning lane. Wanting to edge my way over to the correct lane, I carefully looked into my rearview mirror to be sure I could move safely. I systematically made my way into the next lane. At least, that's how I remember it.

But my brother-in-law tells another version of that tale, and his seems to hold more weight. He was stopped at the same intersection by the lights and saw the entire incident as it unfolded. *That idiot is going to cause an accident!*

As he retold the story later, it was peak-hour traffic—around five-thirty in the afternoon—when he sat at the light. He couldn't believe his eyes. A driver had made a big, sweeping U-turn, darting across three lanes of traffic to reach the turning lane. He recognized the passenger as the preacher's wife—with her arms over her head. He had a sneaking suspicion...sure enough, the pieces quickly came together when he saw his wife's old, olive green Torino. He shook his head and laughed. *Oh no. That's my sister-in-law, Amy!*

He told the story—as a rite of initiation—to all my future dates after our first family dinner. "Let me tell you something about this girl you're going out with. I think you better know what you're getting yourself into."

"Please," I begged, "Stop telling that story!"

At twenty-three, that one incident destroyed my future relationships. Is it any wonder I married out of the country? I wasn't sure which was worse—submitting an insurance claim or sitting through the story.

I had no idea why I drove so poorly, but I never gave up. That's probably why the accidents kept happening. I was too embarrassed to say I wasn't comfortable driving, least of all in downtown Erie, but driving was part of my job.

On a typical work day in our Catholic Charities immigration office, my supervisor asked me to drive two newly-arrived, Hungarian refugees to the Health Department for their required TB shots. I started to sweat. The problem was, I didn't know where it was and I wasn't familiar with the new agency car. But I got directions, and the three of us set out.

"We arrive into country today morning. We see airport only," said Hórvat, the taller of the two.

"Oh, how nice," I chattered. "Welcome to Erie!" *Turn here. No, that's a one-way street.* I skidded to a halt. "Just a little drive," I said with a smile as I made another wrong turn.

Finally, I pulled into the driveway. "Here we are," I said, poking the nose of the car into the drive, starting and stopping until I was certain I was off the crowded street. I finally let out a deep breath. *Made it.*

I buzzed us into the Health Department and my normal confidence returned. Together, we filled out their forms and they received their shots. One refugee couldn't stop talking, but the other couldn't find his voice. I put his silence down to the newness of the surrounding area, lack of sleep and perhaps the painful injection. It couldn't have been the long nervous trek across town.

Too soon we headed back to the car. Zoltan, the quiet one, patted the seat behind him several times. *What's he looking for? Did he forget something? Maybe his wallet?*

I wrinkled my nose. "Money?" I asked, taking out a dollar bill to show him and pointing to the brick building. "Forget?"

"No, no, no. Car." He turned a stricken face to the other fellow and spoke in his native language.

The more communicative Hórvat clarified the problem. "He want cloth. Belto," he said, pulling on an imaginary seatbelt to demonstrate.

After everyone was belted in, I prepared to back out. I swear someone must have shifted my side mirror, because when I took a glance at the traffic, I didn't see the other car at the edge of the driveway. But there was no mistaking what we all heard—the crunch of metal against metal.

73

After all that careful driving, I had my first work accident.

When I looked over to reassure my passengers everything was under control, Zoltan, the silent bearded Hungarian, had covered his eyes, scrunched up his shoulders and was shaking as he whispered to himself. I guessed that was Hungarian for "I escaped the terror in my country only to come to America and find this."

I didn't know what to say and didn't think "Welcome to America!" with a bright smile, or "How is your arm now?" were the best choice of words. Maybe he needed a glass of strong Pálinka.

When I returned to the office and haltingly explained the mishap, my unmoved supervisor grabbed the keys and scolded me. "The new car! Sister Theresa will not be happy. We'll have to—"

"I know," I finished glumly, "turn the claim into the agency's insurance."

At my end-of-year review, my supervisor held that tiny offense against me and she let me go. Another boo-boo in the line-up of Amy's mishaps.

*****

Whenever it was time to renew my driver's license, I always sent in the registration the same day I received the form in the mail. When I received the official camera card, I drove to the Department of Motor Vehicles to take an up-to-date photo for my new license so it would be good for the next four years. That was how I kept my license current even when I lived overseas.

When I was diagnosed with RP at the age of twenty-eight, I finally understood why I was accident-prone, and limited my driving to going to work and back, and doing errands around town. Most of the time, I lived overseas where most people used the public transport system. In 1997, on my last teaching stint abroad, I lived in a village near the desert. Most expatriates who lived there bought large, four-wheel drive vehicles. That was when I finally stopped driving.

But I kept renewing my license. Choosing to give up a driver's license is one of the most terrifying hurdles for anyone losing vision. The psychological impact of no longer driving can be worse than the vision loss itself. It means giving up freedom.

In many cultures, especially western societies, driving is the key to independence. Those who surrender their driver's license, even people who say, "It's the responsible thing to do," heavily feel the loss. Giving up my license meant a head-on collision with my pride.

After moving back to the United States, though I hadn't actively driven for ten years, I went through a series of phases—pretending to look for a car, not finding the right one, not having a place to park it, losing interest in the search and finally opting for walking as a healthy alternative mode of exercise—rather than tell people I was losing my vision. It wasn't until I started orientation and mobility training that these pretenses eased to a halt and I could admit to others I didn't drive anymore.

Yet I kept my license. I gripped it as tightly as a security blanket to reassure myself I was like everyone else—even though I no longer sat behind the wheel. Carrying my driver's license made me feel more independent. I guess that was part of my denial.

A few years ago, I walked into the Department of Motor Vehicles with my white cane to renew my license once again. I must have looked ridiculous as I swept my way to the counter. I figured they'd decline the renewal when they saw my cane, and I prepared myself for the worst.

"Sorry, I do have my camera card here. But I'm kind of late in renewing my license this time," I said with downcast eyes. Ten months overdue was more than late. That, in itself, was grounds for the sit-down-you'll-have-to-take-another-test speech. Of course, I would have never passed either the eye exam or the driver's test.

"Oh no, that doesn't matter," the clerk said. "Go to that man in the next room and he'll take your photo."

I looked in the direction he pointed. "Oh. Okay," I said, hardly able to believe my luck.

The usual crowd of sixteen-year-olds must have been somewhere buying school clothes or attending last-minute parties at the beach. The place seemed eerily silent—no lines, no crying babies, no distraught parents. No one else but me. No witnesses.

In the adjoining room, the clerk sat at a small desk. I tentatively swept my cane over to him. "Excuse me. I need my photo ID taken. Is this the right place?"

He mumbled something, probably, "Are you crazy?" I wouldn't have blamed him. There I stood with my cane, asking to get my photo taken for my *driver's* license.

I hesitated, then took a seat in the empty waiting room.

The first clerk scurried in. "This man can take care of you," he said, pointing to the clerk, "I should have told you exactly where to go."

The man scowled at me. "Gimme your card."

I handed over my camera card and wondered why he hadn't noticed my cane. Or was he surly because he *did* notice it? Maybe he was just a grouch. I smiled nervously, unsure of myself.

The man jutted out his chin to a chair behind me. "Sit down." He picked up a camera lens and fiddled with the settings.

I sat down, holding my cane awkwardly in my hand. Feeling uncomfortable, I folded the cane in half and set it at my feet, seconds before the camera clicked.

"Pick the best one," I told the clerk. Without interest, he selected one. Afterward, he told me to write my signature on a small screen. A moment later, I held my driver's license in my hand.

"Thank you," I breathed, as I swept my cane smoothly across the floor, admiring my brand new beautiful driver's license in my other hand.

"Let me get the door for you," the first clerk offered, as friendly as could be.

"Sure, thanks."

I stepped out of the Department of Motor Vehicles with a smile on my face. I paused and waved my driver's license in front of me for everyone to admire, feeling like a beauty queen gesturing to my adoring fans. Only I don't think these folks were adoring. Or even fans.

Cars screeched to a halt. Those passing by pointed. A young teenager took a photo with her cell phone. It didn't matter. I waved it at everyone. As I reached the car, I folded up my cane and entered, still beaming.

"Didn't they make you get an ID card instead?" my brother asked.

"Nope. He-e-ere's…my driver's license!"

My brother's eyes widened as he took it out of my hands and examined it. "They're blinder than you are!"

I shrugged. At least I still had my driver's license.

"Wait a minute! They hire vision-impaired employees to take photo IDs. Remember I mentioned this to you months ago when you were trying to find work?"

"Yes, I *do* remember."

Some call it divine justice, I call it *blind* justice. However it happened, it worked for me. I was safe for another four years.

I do know why having a driver's license instead of a photo ID is such a big deal. When someone asks for ID, the first thing people reach for is their driver's license. If I don't have one, it's almost like giving up part of my personal identity—the last vestiges of my independence—the part that stubbornly remains in denial.

But I know my independence comes from the inside. It isn't linked to a symbolic license I don't use, and I never have to worry about another insurance claim. My freedom stretches out in front of me, a long tree-lined road filled with security and new perceptions of my worth I never fully realized.

16/ "MAY I HAVE THE FLOOR, PLEASE?"

Sometimes I make up stories to help me move past my challenges when I can't see things clearly. Because I have to think of split-second explanations, these fabrications can be fairly weak. But I just have to go with them, as was the case on an overnight trip when I tried to orient myself to a stranger's home.

I slammed the car door, swung my travel bag over one shoulder and picked up my cane. Squinting—seemed like the shades I wore hardly cut the glare of the evening sun—I stopped and waited for Steve, a fellow author.

"Where to, Steve?" As I waited for his response, I blinked several times to help my eyes adjust faster to the brightness outside the car.

"Straight ahead."

I swept my cane forward, and a minute later, it came up against stairs.

Steve let out a long sigh. "I'm right behind you. Go on in." Clearly our long day had taken a toll on him too.

Why didn't he go before me? It was *his* friend's house and *he'd* made the arrangements. He probably thought he was being a gentleman by having me go first.

At the top step, I heard a voice say, "Come in, dear."

I braced myself for the inevitable change in lighting—again. As a matter of habit, I removed my sunglasses and perched them on my head as I moved out of the way to let Steve in. It was like stepping into a dark movie theater after the show started. I hated that.

The dim lighting cast a pale arc in the room. I stood still, and let the room come into focus. Steve introduced me to Rita.

What I can see varies. Sometimes it's all a blur. Other times I have no idea what is next to me yet I may see something far away clearly. Because I still have some of my central vision, I can usually see objects—like the computer screen or a person's features—in great detail, but everything around them is blurry. It depends on how much my brain fills in the missing parts for me.

That day, I could see the face of Steve's friend, Rita. She had sharp features, but when she leaned my way, they softened with her smile. She wore her hair pulled back in a simple ponytail and lounged in what looked like a floor-length caftan. I held out my hand first to avoid the she-wants-to-shake-your-hand moment. Our brief hand clasp surprised me.

She squeezed my hand so hard, she left an imprint on my palm.

Rita seemed to move around quickly. Her voice came from different parts of the room. My eyes darted back and forth trying to keep up with the talk between Steve and Rita.

Finally, she said, "Let me show you where you'll be sleeping."

I straightened from where I was leaning against the wall. Either my eyes took longer than normal to adjust or the room was unusually dim.

Why don't people turn on more lights?

I unfolded my cane, ready to move. Rita was right next to me. I could see her eyes fixed on my cane.

"Steve, close the basement door," she barked. "All we need is for her to fall down the stairs."

For *her* to fall down the stairs? Did she mean *me?* I wanted to remind her I *can* hear.

"Excuse me." Steve pushed past me, and I heard a door close. "Just to let you know," Steve warned, "Rita's on oxygen. Don't trip on her tube."

I gulped. I could see Rita's face and her clothing but not even a glimpse of a thin, clear oxygen line. I looked down. Where was it? *Oh Lord, please don't let me step on it!* "Um, Steve, where exactly is…."

I froze, terrified of tripping over her tubing or getting my cane tangled up in it. *Where did Steve go?* I heard him say from somewhere across the room, "You okay?"

You'd think after delivering a bomb like that he'd take my arm and guide me. But no, I heard Steve unzipping his suitcase and from the silence, guessed he was busy digging through his clothes.

Rita yawned loudly. "Come along, dear."

My heart thudded so hard I could actually hear it. Best not to use my cane. I folded it up, trying to steady my trembling fingers as I stretched the elastic around the cane to secure it, and took hesitant baby steps after Rita, careful to keep my distance. I couldn't see where the walls were. My eyes latched onto the bright red and yellow in her caftan and clung to it as if it were a flashlight.

At the end of the hallway, Rita entered a room. She leaned in and switched on a small table lamp. "I'll let you get settled. If you need anything, or have any questions, just give me a shout," she said as she left.

I set my bag and cane down. For just a moment, I imagined myself shouting, "Hey Rita, just one question. Did you pay the electric bill last month?"

Maybe the darkness kept her cool, and she could breathe better. But I didn't dare ask her that. Too personal. She might feel obligated to turn on the lights, and that might not be healthy for her.

I sat on my bed, but knew I had to leave the room…sometime.

Finally, I picked up my cane and headed back. As soon as I entered the living room, I folded the cane up again, feeling awkward. I could see absolutely no furniture—which was crazy. I knew there had to be furniture throughout the room. What living room doesn't have furnishings? The sun had set, so no help there. And there was only one ceiling light on.

I wanted to scream, "Help! Help! Where's the furniture? Invisible! Gone!"

What I did was fluff up my hair, throw my silk scarf over one shoulder and lean down toward the weak light beaming onto the rug. I swept my hand over it as if it were the plush carpet in a Fifth Avenue hotel. "Dah-ling, I love a good cah-pet!" I sat down, stretched out, crossed my ankles and sighed, as if I had arrived.

The red and yellow caftan seemed to shrink away from me. Had Rita backed up?

"Well, I've not had that reaction to my living room carpet before. It was a Sears special. If you feel that way about my carpet, wait until you try my chair." She tried to make it sound inviting, but I wasn't buying it.

My response?

Not, "Where is it?"

Not, "Gladly, if I could only see it."

Nope, instead I said, "I prefer this lovely spot right where I am. After being on my feet all day, it's luxurious to stre-e-e-tch out now like this." I wiggled my toes in ecstasy.

Rita put a hand to her throat and coughed. I patted the space around the floor with my fingertips. Was her tubing under one of my feet? No. Phew!

She said, "Oh, very well, dear, as you wish," her voice light and, I suspect, teetering on disbelief.

All this because I couldn't ask for help to find her chairs or *any* of her furniture. It was really quite ridiculous, this pretense. Don't get me wrong; I liked a good carpet as much as the next guy, maybe even more. But I did feel a bit odd seated in the middle of the floor while my two adult counterparts sat nicely on the cushions of their respective chairs. I wasn't the Great and Powerful Wizard of Oz. More like the Great Pretender.

Once I declared how much I loved sitting on the floor—practically screaming out my exotic fondness for carpet threads—I felt obligated to continue my charade and love of all places low.

Rita turned to Steve. "Do you think she'd like some wine? That's what I'm having."

"I'll get a beer for myself," Steve said, standing up. "Amy will have some bottled water. She doesn't 'do' wine."

I don't? Hello. I can hear this conversation and I can speak for myself. I wanted to say, "Don't you think someone who loves a fine carpet would equally love a fine wine?" But I kept silent and instead, drank my fine water in a wine-stem glass.

"Are you sure you don't want to sit on a chair?" Rita asked once.

"Oh n-o-o, and give up all this comfort? Not a chance!" I leaned back and patted the carpet as if it were a pillowed cloud. I smiled as if there were no better.

Steve grumbled, "If she prefers the floor, as she obviously does, let her lie in comfort. We've had a long day trying to sell our books."

Once I planted myself on that carpet, I feared moving within the darkness, even to find a comfy chair. Funny how a clear little piece of tubing could put me in such a dither. Why didn't I just *say* something?

As I sipped my spring water and listened to the two of them ramble on about their past, the need for sleep caused me to be bold. "I'll head off to bed, if you don't mind."

"Steve! Did you close the basement door?"

"Yes, I did. I did. I did."

Again, I took out my cane and made my way to my assigned bedroom, where I finally relaxed.

The next morning, on the way to the bathroom, it happened. I stepped on Rita's oxygen cord and I didn't even realize it.

Rita stopped in her tracks. "My life line...." she said, lifting a hand to her throat and giving a slight cough. I stared, gasping as it became clear what I'd done. I could feel the thin tubing under one toe. I removed my foot and let the air stream flow unrestricted to poor Rita just as she took matters into her own hands. She picked me up and moved me to the right.

"Oh, Rita! I'm *so* sorry."

"No, it happens." She coughed again. "My grandkids step on it all the time."

"Oh." And they could see.

Both of us survived that ordeal, and we didn't even let it stop us. In the bathroom, she gestured to a stack of towels. "If you want to take a shower...."

I fumbled around for a minute and set my clothes down. "Rita, which is the hot and which is...." I stopped, looked around and couldn't see anyone. She'd vanished. People seemed to leave without my knowing it. She probably excused herself, and I didn't see her go.

A minute later, Rita tapped on the bathroom door. "Something hot to drink?"

"Ah, sure, if it's no trouble," I said, deciding not to take the shower.

After a quick cup of vanilla herbal tea and a look at her photo album in the stronger morning light, Steve said, "Thanks for the hospitality. We need to get on the road."

Breathing a sigh of relief, I stood up. "I'll just get my bag."

"Hang on. Steve, check that basement door!"

I heard him move to my right and rattle the doorknob. "Closed, Rita."

Now that I had an idea where it was, I rolled my eyes and swept right past that dratted basement door.

After we said our goodbyes, Steve and I chatted on the long drive home about his friendship with Rita. In the lull that followed, I thought about the situation I'd faced. For most people, going to a new place wasn't a big deal. They could see where they were going. They could pick out the bathroom, the hallway or a chair and find where to turn on the lamps.

Completely blind people might scoff at me. They had to adjust with no light at all. I was amazed at their ability to do so. But for me, gradually losing my vision and learning how to be blind, orienting myself to a new and very dark place was not an easy feat. Throw in other monkey wrenches like pride and an oxygen line, and you've got one Great Pretender. My inner dialogue kept repeating, *I want to go home. I want to go home. There's no place like home.*

Like me, Dorothy found herself in an unfamiliar environment. She wasn't at all comfortable in the world of munchkins, the yellow brick road and a wicked witch trying to steal her ruby slippers. She just wanted to get back to the familiar—home.

Suddenly I laughed, right there in the car. Like Dorothy and her ruby slippers, I had had what I needed—my cane.

The irony floored me. Why hadn't I used it to better discover my surroundings inside the house all along? With my cane, I could have found the chair, the sofa or an end table. That's why I had a cane. But I set it aside, forgetting I had the power from the start. Instead, I pretended to be in control.

Why did I do that? Fear, of course.

But Rita had fears, too. She had probably never interacted with a vision-impaired person before. She didn't want me anywhere near that basement door. All she could hear in her mind was the *thunk-thunk* of me hitting each step and ending up with a broken arm or leg. Maybe she feared being sued. Most of the time, Rita was afraid to directly speak to me.

We both let our fears get the better of us. She was just as much in the dark to know how to handle the situation as I was. She couldn't bring herself to ask how much vision I had. She didn't want to offend, or admit or share. Just like me.

The more I thought about it, the more I realized that it didn't matter if a person were vision-impaired or sighted. We needed to embrace moments of challenge and let go of that semblance of control.

If we choose to, we can use the tools we already have to step into the light of honesty.

17/ THE NON-EXISTENT DOOR

"May I help you?" The voice of the receptionist at the optometrist's office sounded sharp, almost alarmed.

I dropped my hand down to my side. "There isn't another door, is there?"

"Pardon me?"

She must have spied my cane then because her voice softened, though it still held a hint of amusement. "Not that I've ever seen."

Too late, I pointed to the entrance. "That's the only door in the office, right?" I had been pushing against the air, trying to find the door handle to an inner door to the office. I rolled my eyes and extended my cane again. The tip hit at something hard. "I'm at the front desk, aren't I?"

"Yes, you are."

Oh, great. Not exactly the impression I wanted to begin today's marketing attempt with.

Now that my eyes had adjusted to the interior lighting, and things came into slightly better focus, I introduced myself and said I was the author of the book I was holding. "Is the low-vision specialist here today?"

"She's with a patient now."

I groaned. Who knew how long that would be? I had someone waiting for me in the car who had limited time this morning.

"Do you know how long…."

"No, ma'am."

I launched into a quick Plan B. "How about I leave my book with you to give to her? I'll write a note explaining my proposal."

The receptionist handed me a paper and pen. If she thought it strange that I could write but not see well, she didn't let on.

I wrote my message, being sure to leave my contact information in it. Perhaps she would call this very afternoon to say, "Yes, I'd be thrilled to review your book." In small towns, people helped each other.

I breathed a silent prayer and gave the woman my penned message.

"The door is straight ahead about six feet. The handle is on the left."

"Got it!" I turned and walked across the office. This time when I pushed, my hand met with a solid handle and a real door swung open. I walked out, my head high and my cane in front.

Funny how coming into a new place is so challenging, while leaving is a whole lot easier. I wonder if that's why we hesitate when pursuing our goals. There are no instructions. We just take our chances and guess at what is there. As clarity comes, we quickly meet the challenge with any given resource. Knowing we took that hesitant step is confidence-building. Others take their cue from us and guide us on our way.

No one knows exactly where the doors are. We all have to push until we come up against one that really moves.

18/ SO CLOSE...AND YET SO FAR

I wore my lightweight shorts, a T-shirt and my darkest sunglasses. I tugged on a loose shoelace to tighten it and stood up. "I'll be back soon."

My mother looked up from her book. She frowned. "You're not going running now, are you? Did you forget we're going to the Greek Festival around three o'clock?"

"No, no, no." I tapped the knob on my talking watch. A quarter to two. "I'll be back in time. I just want to get in a quick run."

"I don't know...." She looked pointedly at the clock above the TV. "You lose track of time."

After reassuring her I wouldn't be late, I took off—purposely leaving my cane at home. It didn't do me any good folded up at the entrance to the track. I didn't run with it. Using it to get to the track and back home only reminded me of my limitations and slowed me down. It put me out of the zone. Since I ran every day, the route was engraved in my mind. I knew exactly which sidewalk squares could trip me up. It was a straight shot from my house and took only ten minutes to get there. Running was the only activity to which I refused to take my cane.

I ducked through the gap between two chain-linked fences to get to the track. For the first couple of minutes I stretched—if you could call what I do stretching. I like to think I'm a running machine with muscles like rubber bands. The truth is, at my age, my stretching ends just below my knees. I set the timer on my cell phone to beep in half an hour, then slipped it back into the passport-sized zippered bag I wore around my neck.

Ready.

The sun warmed my face and I ran like the wind. Well, a gentle breeze. Bold white lines helped me stay in the correct lane. The third lane was my favorite, and unless another runner was using the track, I always chose it. The starting line didn't seem so far away. Four laps were a mile. If it was a good day, I'd get in a mile and a half.

I found my rhythm and liked the gentle thump my feet made as they hit the pavement. By my third lap, I was sweating so much my sunglasses slid down my nose. It slowed me down to have to adjust them, so I crinkled my nose to push them up—like nose calisthenics—and kept on running.

Not a single cloud in the sky. As I rounded another curve, I looked down and found myself in one of the outer lanes. *Here I go, running cockeyed again.* With a firm set to my lips, I crossed back into my preferred lane. Fifth lap. Nearing the starting-lane marker, I slowed down and switched directions to prevent the backs of my legs from getting sunburned. I was halfway around the track when I crashed into one of the hurdles used by the track team.

I staggered forward, rubbing my hip. Something happens every time I change directions. It's my eyes. They probably pick up obstacles on only one side. If I come at something from another direction, I am more apt to miss it.

What time is it? Two minutes to go. Let me just finish this lap. Do I have time for another?

I decided against it, which was a good thing because it took longer than I thought to finish. I still had a fourth of the way to go when my alarm went off. I fished it out of my bag and silenced it. *Gotta hurry!* I did my cool down and went through the motions of stretching.

"The time is two thirty-nine," the toneless, electronic voice of my watch announced when I pressed the button.

Cutting it short here. I better start home.

I left the track. Passed the bleachers. Headed across the grass for the chain-linked fence. Funny how I couldn't manage a straight line. I meandered from clover to clover as I tried to get my bearings. Hoped no one was watching.

Where is that entrance?

A sharp pain pricked my leg. Cringing, I jerked away. Had I rubbed up against some ant colony in the higher grass? I had a history of run-ins with ants. While I hopped around like a lunatic, it occurred to me that ant colonies are found in mounds of dirt and not grass. I stopped slapping at the imaginary ants. Probably a bee sting. Something got me for sure.

Where was the opening? I had to get home.

I squinted. Maybe that was it, but the fence didn't seem in the right place. I shouldn't be seeing all this open space. And too dark-colored. I took a few hesitant steps forward. My eyes swept over the area, trying to grasp onto something familiar. I saw something green. I had veered off toward the tennis court.

What time was it?

I turned around and re-oriented myself. As I locked my eyes on the entrance, I moved sideways to keep it within my view. I held out my hand—exactly as I would have with my cane—and finally felt the chain links under my fingertips. I curled them over the sharp wires so as not to bump or scrape my head.

Instead of turning left at the blacktop, I started off in the opposite direction. No big deal, I decided when I realized my error. I could get home that way too. Just a matter of following a square plan. I reviewed it in my head. *At the first cross street, take a right. Follow the school on the same side of the street. When the school property ends, it's another right. Keep going until the end of the road. Cross it. Then a left. Two blocks. Home sweet home.*

A simple square.

I checked my time again. "Two forty-two."

I can make it. It's only a couple of minutes' walk. I can do it.

This called for speed. I half-skipped, half-walked on the blacktop. My right foot came across some bars, and I dipped down. Stopped. *What was that? A drain. Now I see it. Just a drain.*

The pavement inclined slightly. *The Middle School should be on the right. There it is.*

I turned right. *A piece of cake from here.* I walked faster—past the construction area, which I could tell by the green-netted drop cloths set up to mask the disarray and the big utility bin inside the fence. *That smell—wet cement!* I gagged. Pinched my nostrils shut and scurried past the workers. Once past the area, the smell receded. I breathed deeply and continued on my way.

One more block. I passed Mrs. Minskevitch's old farmhouse. She hadn't lived there in decades, but I still called it her house.

At the corner, the familiar street sign rose like a solid sentry. Only one tiny problem. With sunglasses on, the shadows clouded my vision, but with them off, the sun blinded me. I couldn't read the sign either way. Never a perfect medium. But this had to be my turn-off.

Two turns down, one to go.

I started out moving fast. Then slowed down. *What's the name of this street? I should be nearing the red brick house. Was that on Riley or Miles Ave? I grew up around here. I should know this street. Could be further up. Is this the route? Wait. No. Yes. This has to be correct.*

Sweat crept up the side of my neck, and my T-shirt chafed under my armpits. I plucked the shirt away to give myself air and swiped my hand across the back of my neck. With the palm of my hand, I wiped sweat on the front of my running shorts.

The neighborhood was quiet. Peaceful. Everything in order. Flowers waved gently in the breeze. A dog of some unknown breed ran out to investigate me. Apparently I didn't pose a big enough threat because it retreated without a growl or even a bark. I heard the thrum of a loud engine and saw an older man riding a lawn mower. I would ask him. Before I gathered up the courage, the form disappeared behind the side of the house. Just as well. What if the man knew my family? Would he think I suffered from early onset dementia?

See, you think you know so much and you chose not to bring your cane.

I ignored that inner dialogue and kept walking.

Removing my sunglasses to see better, I squinted into the sun. Lynn's parents should live on the corner house of...maybe...this street. Where was the wheelchair ramp? But if this were the house, where were the two front trees that were supposed to be there? Or were they bushes?

Two female voices caught my attention. I whipped around in their general direction, but heard only the whiz of pedals passing me. Moments later, I saw backs bent over their bikes—probably no less than twenty-one gears these days—and then their voices, too, vanished.

My shoulders slumped. Everyone seemed full of purpose. I was the only one out of place in this picture-perfect neighborhood.

If a driver came my way, I'd stop and ask where I was. *Come on, cars! Where are you?*

Just my luck. The roads were empty. Leaves on the shade trees didn't even stir on the sidewalk. *On the sidewalk?* I was on the *road*, on the lookout for the next set of signs plunked at the corner of some grassy lot. *I'd better get out of the road!*

The heat beat down. I bit my bottom lip. Jutted my head. Stopped. Backtracked. There it was—Riley and Miles. Okay, I was on Miles Avenue. I stopped to think for a moment. Did Riley or Miles come out at the brick house?

I'm gonna be late. I'm gonna be late!

Suddenly, an idea came to me. I took out my iPhone and read my address into the phone. "Take me home, Siri."

Siri gave me instructions. "Go ten feet southwest...."

I guessed as to which direction was southwest, and sure enough, there was Lynn's parents' house. I laughed when I noticed the trees I remembered turned out to be a row of bushes. That didn't matter. I knew where I was. Before long, I arrived at the red brick house. Relief flooded into me as I crossed onto my street and broke into a sprint. When I neared home, Siri let me know I was approaching my destination.

I slipped in through my garage door. My cell phone rang halfway up the stairs to my apartment. I reached for it and put it on speaker phone.

It was Mom. "Are you ready to go to the Greek Festival?"

"Yeah." If I sounded out of breath, Mom didn't say anything. "I'll meet you down at the car."

I made it. Talk about a close shave! I headed back down the stairs, reaching for my cane at the door. In the crowd at the Greek Festival, this stick would make all the difference. I had had enough excitement for one day.

Being partially sighted is confusing. Some things look familiar from certain angles, but when I come closer, I find my eyes often trick me. What does my brain fill in, and what do I really see? What part does my memory serve me? It's a brain teaser that could wear me down. But I don't let it.

Getting lost in my own neighborhood sure gave me a start. Oh, the irony of successfully traveling the world and yet getting lost a few streets from my home....

19/ STRANGE TESTS

I stared at my computer. "Not the blue screen of death."

The deadline! Was it out of reach? The promised paycheck dissolved before my eyes. In spite of the hot July sun streaming through the window, my hands felt clammy. Had I saved last night's writing? *Please let me have saved it.* What would I do?

A section I had reworked several times had finally come together the night before, but my cell phone had said it was after three in the morning. Time to call it a night. Through sleep-deprived eyes, I had slid my chair away from the desk and groped my way into my bedroom before I sunk into my flowered sheets and a dreamless sleep. The plan was to finish my piece in the morning.

Turning the computer off and rebooting it only brought more alarming news: "Irrecoverable error. Initiating a physical dump to protect blah-blah-blah. For assistance, call your system administrator."

I was a freelance writer, not a business with a plethora of technicians on hand to straighten out my dying system. A quick look at my watch said my nephew-in-law had arrived at work and would be tending to his clients' computer issues.

I called our local computer company, but no one picked up. Their name, B & D Computers, might as well have stood for 'What's the Big Deal' Computers. At nine in the morning, they should answer.

A black computer screen faced me. The precious, hard-fought words to my story were trapped in the inky database.

The owners of B & D Computers occasionally made home calls to troubleshoot, but their tech-savvy knowledge came at a high price. Still, I needed those words, and it would be worth it.

As I waited for a callback from the experts, I phoned my friend, Cat, to vent. "I had such good intentions to finish this morning," I groaned.

"I hear ya' girl. Come on, get out of the house. Don't stew at home over your broken computer. Wash your sorrows away with a coke and chow down on a burger."

"Maybe you're right," I agreed. "Sitting at home and doing nothing is driving me nuts."

"You can always take a pad of paper and write longhand," she reminded. "But I know how you feel. I'll be by to pick you up at noon."

We texted back and forth to decide where to go. "It'll have to be a

McD's day," Cat finally said, "We're busy in the shop today."

At noon, she pulled up in the back driveway and beeped.

When I opened the door, she immediately asked, "Where's your cane? Do you have it with you?"

"Yeah, yeah, yeah." I tapped my canvas bag. "In here."

She waited for me to buckle my seatbelt. "Doesn't do you any good tucked away in your purse. You need to take that baby out and use it," she said lightly.

"I know."

Cat also believed in turning on car headlights in daylight. She said it was safer. She pursued caution. Cat often reminded me not to be careless on a number of issues. In fact, if it were her, she would have saved the document without second thoughts. Why couldn't I remember such things?

"It's just a matter of making it a habit," Cat declared. "Every time you leave the house, use your cane."

"I can see better during the day," I explained, "so I don't always need it."

"Well, didn't your mobility instructor say that, even when *you* can see all right, a cane alerts others to the fact you have sight issues? Remember, they'll be more tolerant if you run into them."

"He did say that." She was catching me on everything today.

After leaving Cat's car, I unfolded my cane and swept my way to the door of the restaurant, where I reached for the handle and went through. "See? Using it."

Cat smiled. "That's why you have it." She picked up a single tray from the counter, holding both our meals. She handed me a couple of napkins and a straw, along with some ketchup. "By the window okay?"

I hung my purse on the back of the chair and had just started to sit down when Cat said, "Not there. The table's dirty. See, there's some mustard. Why don't we sit here instead?" she suggested, setting the tray down on the table next to it.

"Oh. Okay." Leaning my cane against the wall, I hung my purse on the back of the new chair.

I fiddled with the lid of the fruit salad, trying to open it.

"Need some help?"

"Nope, got it." I replied, spilling out some of the contents as I wrestled the lid off.

Cat handed me a strawberry. "Well, what are your options? We use B & D at the shop. It costs about a hundred bucks if they come to you. Why don't you just disconnect your computer and take it to them. That'll save you some money."

She didn't understand the complicated set-up I had with the laptop doing the processing for a second computer's larger screen and keyboard. There were wires everywhere, and I didn't know how to reconnect everything.

"Can you use a laptop? I can loan you mine," Cat offered.

I buoyed on a wave of hope and then took a nosedive as waves of despair engulfed me. Who was I kidding? The print was so tiny on a laptop I once borrowed, it took me two hours to access my email. Cat's keyboard would be too small to see too. But if by some miracle I recalled my password to Dropbox—and that would be a big 'if'—to access my document, how could I work on it? The background wouldn't give me enough contrast. It was like looking at tiny yellow hieroglyphics on a black background. I needed a computer tailored to my vision needs in order to really get any work done.

I explained the challenges to Cat, "...and the cursor and font are too hard to see."

"Make them larger. There's a way you can do it. I'll find out and get back to you on how to do it."

She really wanted to help me, I could tell.

"Yeah, sure, I'd love to borrow it. Thanks for offering."

With a temporary solution hashed out, we left. I hummed, thinking maybe a miracle would find me, and I could hammer out a conclusion to the story even if I didn't have the beginning.

We had almost reached Cat's car when a man called out to me, "Miss, you forgot your cane."

"Oh, thank you, sir." I turned around, intending to recover the forgotten tool.

"I'll wait in the car," Cat said, closing the gap to her vehicle.

When I neared the entrance, the little old man who brought my forgetfulness to my attention said, "I'll get it." He slipped through the glass doors.

I stood, one foot on the sidewalk and the other on the pavement. *Everyone is so helpful. Either they open the door or move aside to let me pass. Now look, this nice guy went to fetch my cane.* These kinds of blessings were the flip side to losing my vision.

The elderly gentleman opened the glass door and extended his arm, cane in hand. I reached for it, but to my surprise, the gentleman held tightly onto it. Instead, he tilted his head and made a funny face.

What an odd little man.

He tilted his head in the opposite direction and made another funny face. He opened and closed his mouth. Watching him contort his face reminded me of my nieces. Sometimes when they take photographs, they pull their lips into hideous frowns. Or they put their fingers in their ears and tilt their heads in an unflattering angle because someone once taught them it was funny.

What was this man *doing?*

Since he hadn't offered me my cane yet, I wasn't sure what to do, so I smiled. His next move was to jut out his head and make his eyes bulge. I continued to watch him. *He must have some mental health issues. Poor guy.* "Thank you for getting my cane," I said cheerfully, reaching out to finally take it.

Although he let go, he moved his fingers back and forth a few inches from my face in a straight line.

I was taken aback. *Best to just ignore his strange behavior.* I smiled once more. "Thanks again. I might have tripped without it." I turned and headed for Cat's car.

In the car, we giggled as I described the eccentric antics of the old chap. Maybe he was senile. Who knew?

A few days later, when I described the situation by phone to my friend, Julio, he said straight away, "He was testing you. He wanted to discover how much you could see."

"What?"

"Sure, I see it all the time on my campus."

I could feel a headache coming on and rubbed my temples. "Just because you have a PhD, you think you know everything. I can assure you that's not what happened. Why would he care how much I can see?" I didn't think that explanation was plausible. The old man seemed senile.

"People want to know what the blind can see. He was testing you."

Was that what the whole finger movement was all about? "Why didn't he just *ask* me?"

"Why didn't you just *tell* him?" Julio was quick to respond. "You're the one who left your cane."

"What business is it of his how much I can or can't see?" I laid my phone down on the counter and crossed my arms.

"It's your duty to educate him. People just want to know. It's no big deal."

"Do you tell people you're not married?"

"We're not talking about me," he reminded. "I'm sure that's what the old man was doing."

By now, I felt certain too, and though I was becoming color blind at this stage of my vision-loss progression, I saw red. It irked me to have someone I didn't know coercing me to reveal the extent of my vision simply to satisfy his curiosity. Unlike the old commercial where someone wonders, does-she-or-doesn't-she (color her hair), this is-she-or-isn't-she (blind) hit me in the gut.

Why was it my duty to educate him? And why did people like the old man insist on knowing how much I could see? It *was* a big deal to me. We all want our privacy, and have a right to choose who and when to share such a sensitive part of ourselves with. If I had known forgetting my cane would have caused such a commotion, I would have definitely left it at home. A cane was supposed to answer questions, not create them.

On the weekend, my nephew-in-law fixed my computer.

"Thank you. My words are now free!" I said, doing a jig. "They aren't trapped anymore in cyberspace." I knew the words I had written weren't really perfect, but they felt like they defined me, and that was good enough for me. I had a distinct voice that moved me forward.

So did using my cane. My computer didn't operate perfectly. The glitches I had to work out took time. Like the ensnared words in cyberspace, my vision was trapped behind an unrecoverable error in the set-up of my eyes. But the beautiful part was that I wasn't dependent on my eyes anymore. I had a back-up, and that operating system worked, though maybe not perfectly. With my cane, I became and remained free.

So having people give me strange tests was simply a glitch, and I didn't need to treat it as the blue screen of death. In fact, I could probably pre-empt any odd behavior by speaking more openly with people about my type of vision loss and its inconsistencies—and by remembering to pick up my cane whenever I exited a building.

20/ THESE NOODLES ARE NOT FOR DINNER

At the end of my Middle East venture, I planned to buy my first house. But my dad talked me out of it. "The wood loft over the garage would make a perfect studio apartment. You'll save yourself a ton of money and still have your own place."

I couldn't resist the offer he made or the unmistakable excitement that crept into his voice as he fleshed out the plans on paper. Dad was never happier than when he was working on a new project.

He put up drywall and transformed the lumber storage area into a cute little apartment that attached to my childhood bedroom and a bathroom. Though I didn't think to ask, he also added several windows to allow more light and enable me to see better.

Dad also cleverly designed a half-wall where my sink and a few cupboards fit nicely. He did the same on the other side of the kitchen for my living room/office. The result: the illusion of a more spacious apartment. A perfect spot for me, Buddy and Midnight, my jet black cat.

Over the opposite side of the steep stairway was a window. From the sink, I could feel the warmth of the sun's rays as they flooded into the apartment. In late afternoon or right after a rainstorm, refreshing cross-breezes between the window and one from the far side of the apartment cooled me.

With the brilliant sun streaming in, I didn't mind washing up after a meal. Where others might have found it tedious, I reveled in creating order from the chaos. The hot, sudsy water seemed almost therapeutic on my hands, and my mind wandered as I washed, rinsed and set the dishes in the strainer.

Finishing up, I wiped a damp dishcloth over my countertops and cupboard doors and reached for the broom. I relished in my favorite chore, sweeping the ceramic tiles.

The tiles' white cloud pattern with its faint hint of blue reminded me of the open sky of the many countries where I'd traveled. Looking down at the floor tiles made me feel as if I were looking into a lake and seeing the sky mirrored on its surface.

I'd catch my breath and recall the words by Azorín José Martínez Ruiz, the nineteenth-century Spanish writer, who in his last act of La Celestina, described the clouds as the sea, both eternal and ephemeral— always the same and yet always changing—so like my vision. I often feel myself grasping for the familiar in my ever-changing environments.

I painted the kitchen walls dark blue and chose the white cupboards myself. It was a chance combination that immediately conjured up memories of Santorini, my favorite Greek island, which had a long tradition of those same vibrant colors—from the white-washed buildings to the dark blue trim around doors and windows. I hung white lace curtains, exactly like those I remembered seeing in the quaint Greek inns where I stayed. With my Mediterranean décor, I felt cocooned in my travel memories, even when my meal plan included the quintessential American cheeseburger, fries and salad.

My office served as the focal point for my creativity—student worksheets, magazine writing and my books. But the kitchen always pulled me back. When I had time, I loved trying out new recipes—foods from the many countries I'd traveled to—or baking some kind of dessert. My favorite was brownies, and I never tired of discovering new variations.

One evening, I decided to attempt yet another recipe from the Internet. This one, fail-proof and mess-free, was my kind of recipe. I had only to melt Baker's Chocolate and butter then add a few other ingredients. When I finished, the batter looked thick and gooey. Oh, what a chocolate-infused aroma filled the kitchen!

I pulled out a rectangular baking dish, tore off a piece of aluminum foil and lightly sprayed it with olive oil. With the foil in the baking dish, I had only to pour the mixture, place it in my pre-heated oven and, *voilà*, fudge-like brownies would emerge. I could hardly wait.

To ensure my ingredients were thoroughly combined, I ran the rubber spatula around the inside of the mixing bowl, which had crept progressively closer to the edge of the counter. In an instant, the bowl tipped. Spun off the edge. I lunged for it. Hoped I could prevent…the grand collision.

But I didn't see the three open drawers, kitty-corner. The silverware drawer smacked me just below my breastbone, taking my breath away. "Oof!" My arm flew out and bumped the bowl. It hit the wall and spiraled down, the force causing the batter to ooze out. The container landed upside-down in the bottom drawer. It seemed like I was in slow motion as I shouted, "Holy Moly."

After recovering from my shock, I surveyed the damage. The sticky mixture splattered on the nearby walls, clinging to utensils in each of the drawers. I saw a glob half the size of my fist on the tile floor, more of it covering the outside hinges of the cupboards and a long trail from the knob of the cupboard door almost to the bottom. There was even some wedged under the stovetop burner.

How could I have forgotten to close the drawers—again? The measuring spoons came from the top drawer, the foil and pot holders from the second and measuring cups from the bottom. Mom always said taking time to look around prevented accidents. *Well, Mom, I'm looking now, and all I can see is a lovely disaster. Mess-free recipe, my eye!*

I'd have to take *everything* out of the drawers, wipe them down and put it all back. After that, I'd need to clean off the countertops and cupboard doors. A lot of hard work, and no brownies to show for it.

I groaned and stumbled over to the breakfast bar to collect myself. Sitting on a tall stool, I rested for a few minutes. My eyes flew open when I felt nibbling on my foot. *What?* It was Buddy, my dog. Always on the lookout for new developments, especially when it came to food, he had quietly made his way over to me and was licking my sock. "Buddy, stop that." *What is he doing?*

Then I noticed footprints leading from the cupboard to the breakfast bar. *Uh-oh, I must have stepped in the big blob by the drawers and tracked it across the floor. Good going, Amy.* I peeled off both socks and tossed them onto the floor. Buddy promptly picked up the chocolate-soiled one and carried it a short distance away.

I checked the clock. It read 21:00 hours. Time to begin "Operation Brownie Recovery." I filled up the dishpan with hot, sudsy water and took out a fresh dishcloth. Then I sponged down the drawers and wiped the entire vicinity with a thoroughness that only comes with the threat of a court martial. My mother was like a general and noticed every spot.

After I finished, I saw a brown smudge on the wall under the breakfast bar. *Oh, I missed that.* When I bent over with the dishcloth, my forehead slammed against the wood. I'd been so intent on the spot, I missed seeing the more obvious countertop. *Whoa.* I rubbed my head. *Ouch, that hurt!* The breakfast bar was in my blind spot—but the brownie smudge was in clear view. The inconsistencies of RP. My eyes traveled down to a soggy sock. Buddy had made that mess.

"Buddy!"

He came lumbering into the kitchen with an innocent expression.

"You bad boy."

He gazed at me lovingly.

"Don't do that. I'm mad at you. Go lay down."

He stretched out in front of the oven, still watching me. It was as if he were saying, "Enough is enough."

A lump the size of a small goose egg had formed on my forehead, and as I rubbed it, I watched Buddy lay his head on the tile. "So you're going to sleep where I want to bake. I give up."

Buddy let out a contented doggie sigh as if he were sure all along I'd see things his way. The no-fail, mess-free brownie concoction had failed on a grand scale, partly because of Buddy, but mostly due to my mobility problems in the kitchen. It has taken several knocks to my head to accept that not only do I need to be watchful as I venture outdoors and somehow prepare myself for unexpected obstacles, I am now at the point in my vision loss where I have to be careful in my most familiar environment.

Dangers lurk everywhere. Not only do I have to be more aware of open drawers and breakfast bars, but harmless walls can stop me cold. If I happen to turn in the wrong direction, in ten seconds I will have a lump the size of Texas on my forehead. A small, plastic stool I use to put away the dishes has to be rotated to different locations or I'll stumble across it, sending it flying to the other end of the room.

Buddy has taken on the full-time job of consoling me, even when he's the cause and I trip over him.

When I questioned my mobility instructor how I could remain safe inside the familiarity of my own home, he demonstrated a defense stance with arms in front. "Find the obstacle with your arms first to avoid a painful head-on collision or anything thigh-high or lower." Whenever I assumed that stance, I felt like an underweight quarterback ready to make a touchdown and lost my concentration. That plan quickly grew tiresome.

"In the house, you can also use a collapsible cane," my instructor informed me.

I agreed to test it out, and a few weeks later, the new cane arrived. This lightweight variation of my other cane slid easily across the tiles and seemed a good compromise—an indoor version of my cane, much like slippers are to shoes.

The doorbell rang one afternoon, and my friend called, "Are you ready to run errands?"

"Yep!" I shouted, grabbing my cane from the corner of the kitchen and racing down the stairs so my driver wouldn't have to wait. I was halfway across the yard when I realized the "cane" felt heavier than normal. I looked down and saw that I was truly sweeping the grass—with a broom and not my cane.

"Hang on, I'll be right there," I called out to Judie in the driveway. In a moment of spontaneity, I held up the broom in both hands as if to test the wind quality. My laughter changed to my best menacing witchy cackle as I said to the broom, "Not today, my pretty!"

I remember my mom saying plenty of times over the years, "Slow down and look at what you're doing." That might work if I could only learn to follow it. I'd catch half the mistakes I never saw.

One day a friend said, "I have a solution for you."

"Really? What?"

"I'm going to bring you some noodles," Melissa said. "Perhaps some blue noodles."

"Noodles?" My eyebrows creased as I tried to figure out how pasta would solve my dilemma.

"Yes, some blue ones," she repeated. "But these noodles are not for dinner." She laughed. "You'll see."

The next time she visited, she carried two foam noodles, the ones used for floating in swimming pools. "This is an RV hack," she crowed, "and I think it's going to work perfectly. Now, let's see if we can fit it to your nasty ol' breakfast bar."

"What's an RV hack?"

"Like a quick, inexpensive solution for those living in RVs—recreational vehicles. My hubby, Larry, is always hitting his head because of the tight quarters in our RV."

"Got it."

Melissa walked her hands over the length of the breakfast bar and repeated the same action to the foam noodle. "This is about the right length." She then cut a narrow slice down the length of the foam and slipped it over the edge of the finished slab of wood. "There. How's that?"

"Well, we'll find out soon enough."

"Now, what about your cupboards?" She measured the doors and then went to work, cutting two small pieces off the lengthy foam noodle and setting the rest aside. She picked up each piece and made a slice halfway through both of them.

I leaned in, impressed by her precision cutting.

"See, we'll put these two foam pieces on the corner of this cupboard door. If you forget and leave the cupboard door open, next time your noggin will hit the foam noodles and not the door itself," she finished with a satisfied smile.

"Oh, good idea!"

I found that her RV hack did indeed help me to some degree.

Sometimes vision-impaired people stay inside because it seems to be safer in a confined, familiar environment. This might be true for someone who had to adjust to complete blindness, but for someone still with some vision, it's like a game of hide-and-seek.

"Gotcha!" the wall shrieks, "You're it!" Or the door I've forgotten and left ajar laughs, "Olly olly in come free!" I know I've been had again.

It is only when I look down at the cloud-like design on the tile floor in my kitchen that I remember Azorín's observations again, stating how the sky and the clouds have witnessed the same passions and the anxieties of mankind for centuries. The clouds are so elusive and yet such a fixture in the sky. He concludes with these words, "*Las nubes, sin embargo, que son siempre distintas en todo momento, todos los días van caminando por el cielo....*" (While clouds, nevertheless, are always distinct in each moment, every day they are walking across the sky.)

The idea, expressed so beautifully in Spanish, describes the continual loss of my sight—a permanent condition that cannot be tied down or stopped, an entity that continually moves forward in time. The fact that clouds never leave the sky is key to my optimism. This encourages me to hang onto the hope that I'll retain some degree of vision for as long as I live. Of one aspect I'm certain—I'll keep discovering new strategies to cope with the changes when I most need them.

21/ HERE WE GO MARCHING

With a quick wave to my housemate, I stepped out of the car. Early commuters sat on the bench under the flickering streetlights, the transit map behind them. Someone pointed, and the bus lumbered into view. They fell into line just as the door opened. Hoisting my teaching bag over my shoulder, I showed the driver my pass and took a seat. Ingram Park Mall became smaller and disappeared altogether as the bus turned toward Loop 410. I settled in for the ride. My stop was last—Lackland Air Force Base.

This time of day no one said much, but come afternoon, Spanglish—a mixture of Spanish and English typical of the southwest—would flow.

We arrived at the main gate before the sun did. A handful of servicemen got off the bus, all dressed in uniform. As a civilian teaching English to the international military, I wore typical teaching attire – with a conservative bent out of respect for the differing roles women play in other cultures.

To make it to the international teaching wing at the west end of the base normally took about twenty minutes at the clip I moved—not too bad considering the darkness, my biggest obstacle. My route included passing headquarters, then the Air Force basic training compound with the early morning recruits out with their squadron, and finally, over to the Defense Language Institute. I looked down so the glare from the streetlights wouldn't throw me off. What would happen if I got turned around? Fortunately, it hadn't happened yet.

I was going over that morning's first lesson in my head when the voice of a training instructor—the TI—blasted through the calm. The airmen's cadence immediately echoed in the still morning. Accustomed to the recruits' early morning regimes, I shouldn't have been startled. As a training base, Lackland served as the funnel for every recruit joining the Air Force. They did basic training in San Antonio and then headed out to their specified training bases.

Traipsing to the Language Lab and back to our classrooms, teachers and students watched trainees go through intricate marching drills, starting in the pre-dawn hours and continuing throughout the day. I sometimes stopped where I was on the sidewalk to watch them pass by. Once I even saw a straggling mismatch of incoming airman before they received their uniforms or had their hair cut.

The TI often shouted his training cadence so loudly, it came through the open classroom windows. Noticing the profanity, we shut the windows—but not before my military students guffawed. I guess there are some military universals shared around the world.

That morning I didn't have time to dwell or admire anyone. The cadence increased in volume. I turned my head to the left, expecting to see them come from their barracks as they usually did. *No group from that direction. Where are they?* The voices I respected so much suddenly sounded...loud. Scary. Threatening. Close. My stomach clenched. My breath came in pants. I froze. I had to move. Somewhere. I turned the corner and immediately realized I'd made a big mistake. There was no sidewalk. Before I could cross the road, they were upon me.

I was engulfed within the group, entangled in the arms and feet of their cadence. Amazingly, no one tripped or slowed down. I felt like a fly being swatted from airman to airman. When they shouted, "Right, right!" I landed left, left. Somehow I got caught in the ninety-degree, precise turns of their steps, and swift-moving knees assaulted me.

I wizened up, changed direction and tried to match my steps with theirs. In short, I had to fit in. So I swung my arms and picked up a few words from the drill sergeant. Every now and again, my voice joined theirs. As I paraded down the street along with the new trainees, it seemed I was a part of that mismatched group from a week earlier.

In step, we turned once. A second quick turn. I inched my way to the outside of the formation until, finally, I freed myself! A few of the less disciplined men at the back turned to stare at me. They doubled over with laughter. One skinny man saluted. Then the column moved forward and out of my view.

For a moment, I stood where I was, too shocked to do anything. The event replayed in my mind. How had that TI missed me? Or had he? Maybe the rule was, don't stop, stay in step unless the TI gave the word.

Pull yourself together. Where was I? Turned around, for sure. A couple of minutes later, I found the nearest crossroads, but it was still too dark to read the sign. Finally, the sun came up, enabling me to figure out how to reach the language part of the training base.

In the parking lot of my building, a student dressed in his country's uniform called out, "Good morning, Mom."

Other privates echoed his greeting. I wasn't his *mother* or *any* of their mothers for that matter. Nervy for someone of that rank. Did I look that old or were they merely homesick?

It didn't hit me until I turned the knob of my classroom door that the students had actually greeted me with the respectful, "Ma'am."

Neither "Mom" nor "Ma'am" aptly described me as I crossed the training base and found myself in the early morning marching cadence on the way to work that day.

Looking back on the situation, when it came to stepping up and owning my diagnosis of Retinitis Pigmentosa, I could relate to those raw recruits best. A year into this disease was nothing. Outwardly, life seemed to stay the same. That morning, it was as if I, too, were inducted in a cadence of marchers with a TI I knew nothing about. I felt exactly like those airmen straight off the plane—scraggly hair, pre-uniform, half-heartedly marching and trying to block out the shouts of their TIs.

Yeah, that was me, mentally. Wide-eyed and clueless.

I had no idea how fast my life would change when I turned the corner of the disease. If I had been prepared, paid a little bit more attention, I would have heard the cadence: "One, two, to the *left*, to the *right*. Lady soldier, grab that flash*light*."

My cane would have been an asset to me then. The recruits have to march with their rifles from the start to get used to handling them. In fact, their TIs want their rifles to become part of their essential gear so they march with them wherever they go. That way, when a recruit needs to use his rifle, he or she instinctively reaches for it. Likewise, if I had handled my cane from the start and viewed it as an essential tool, it would have lost any threat it posed me much later in life. It would have been second nature to use it.

The TIs prepare the recruits to move ahead without question and handle situations smoothly. Oh, to have approached my vision loss systematically, like a disciplined soldier marches in synch with his squadron. If I strain I can faintly hear another far-off cadence: "Sweep to the *left*, sweep to the *right*. Find that *obstacle*. Don't trust your *sight!*"

22/ PARKING LOT AMNESIA

A cane wouldn't have helped me sidestep this event, mostly because in my Texas days, I was galloping past on a horse called denial. Slowing down to a canter might have helped me see the benefits of using a cane. As it was, the scenery just flew on by. One day the sun got in my eyes and I let the reins dangle. It was no surprise when the horse threw me.

*****

It seems like forever ago that I sat behind a wheel and actually drove a car. Boy, did I have a cute little set of wheels—a Plymouth Sundance. In the sunlight, the red paint gleamed. It was the perfect size for me. No need to sit on any pillow with this car.

Dressed in blue jeans and a T-shirt, I set out for the university. Even after living in San Antonio for years, I never tired of being able to leave the house wearing only jeans and a cotton tee in November. Back home, I'd be wrapped in sweaters, a heavy coat, mittens—the whole winter regalia.

With a day off work, I planned to enroll in a graduate program at the San Antonio branch of the University of Texas. UTSA was the buzzword around DLI, the language institute where I taught. The decision to study for my Master's came about abruptly—as most of my choices did. I could move to an island off Japan or stay in San Antonio and spruce up my credentials. I chose the latter.

Slowing down, I switched off the A/C and rolled down the window to let in some fresh air. The radio was set at KXTN-107.5. Country, of course. The sun visor down to help block out the light, I focused on the interchange. Soon I curved around 1604 and followed the tree-lined entrance to the campus.

It wasn't until I turned into the parking lot that I tensed up, clenching my jaw at seeing so many vehicles in the congested area. The car behind mine gave a loud honk. "All right. All right."

Where would I ever park? My fingers gripped the steering wheel while frantically trying to find a spot. I slowly circled the lot, searching for a visitor's space, biting my nails as my eyes darted back and forth. Not a single empty space marked "Visitor." Finally, a spot! This would have to do. *Why didn't I take time to order the parking decal when my acceptance letter came?* I hoped I wouldn't be fined.

"Can you tell me where the admin building is? I'm registering for my classes."

A young Hispanic woman pointed to a flight of steps and I headed off.

The registration process took hours—waiting in various lines, paying here, getting receipts there, returning with ticket stubs. When I finished at four thirty, my shoulders drooped, and I could barely push the door open to leave. Outside, the sudden change in light hit me. Even wearing sunglasses, the glare of the sun made my eyes tear. I blinked several times.

I swung my bag over my shoulder and climbed down some steps, which brought me to the parking area which looked even fuller than before. Where was my car?

In the sea of vehicles, mine seemed invisible. *Not again.*

The wandering began. It went on and on; I felt like a buzzard seeking its prey.

The sun directly overhead didn't help either; it was blinding me. I had to take off my sunglasses to see the cars. *Whoa!* That made it worse. The sun was so intense. In spite of shielding my eyes, they watered like crazy and flew closed.

Meanwhile, where was the car? This was ridiculous. My imagination kicked in. It was the old west. *Where's my horse? I left it grazing along the river's edge, but it must have bolted.* No, a horse would not have the strength to run far in this oppressive heat.

"Ma'am, may I help you?"

I cupped my hand over my eyes. There, right before me, stood a campus policeman.

Yes, officer, my horse wandered away from the San Antonio River, I almost said. "Sorry, um, I have no idea where my car is."

"You are referring to your personal vehicle, Ma'am?"

Sighing, I tried to keep the tears of frustration at bay. "I've been looking for quite a while now."

That darn sun. I rubbed my eyes, but saw a galaxy of black spots. Sounds from around the parking lot filtered in then. People slammed car doors and ran past, heading off to class. They all seemed to know where they were going. I bet they never spent an hour looking for their cars. The sun was really getting to me.

"Ma'am? Ma'am, I'll need some information to help you find your car," the officer repeated.

Like a child reciting her ABCs, I ticked off what I knew. "It's a bright red, four-door Plymouth Sundance. 1990."

His questions seemed to increase in complexity. Which building had I gone in? Which direction did I come from on my return?

I laughed nervously. "Um, I seem to have developed parking lot amnesia."

He stared. "Ma'am, have you been drinking?"

My hands flew to cover flushed cheeks, which surely matched the color of my beloved car. "No, of course not."

After the officer was satisfied with the information I tried to provide, he led the search around the parking lot. Still shielding my eyes from the bright Texan sun, it struck me as ironic that while in search of my "Sundance," the sun took away any desire to dance at all.

It didn't bother me that I was traipsing after the officer, letting him do most of the work while I puzzled over why this kept happening. Yes, not being able to locate my car happened quite often in busy car parks. It wasn't the first time I'd been in a posse to round up my car.

The security policeman searched for another hour or so. He finally said, "Ma'am, are you sure you parked in *this* parking lot?" He sighed. "We have checked every single red vehicle."

Oh no. I wasn't sure at all. "Maybe I parked in another one?"

He mopped the sweat off his brow and said, "Let's check the one on the opposite side of the admin building."

"Yes, good idea."

He took the steps at a fast clip, as only a policeman on a mission could.

I paraded obediently after him, stepping high to keep pace, focusing on the heels of his black shoes—looking away from the sun. We headed up and then down some steps to another crowded parking lot. Ten minutes later, he stopped. "Could this be your red Plymouth Sundance, ma'am?"

"It could be." I cupped my hands over my eyes and peeked at the windshield. Yes, that was my Air Force Base sticker. I wanted to hug the policeman.

But then, seeing my base decal reminded me. *Uh-oh. I never got my campus sticker and the campus security police is standing right beside me.* I backed away from my windshield, thanking him several times.

"Have a good day, Ma'am," the officer said. "Next time pay more attention to where you park."

"And, by the way, I'd get a campus sticker right away if I were you."

23/ WHO WILL LEAD WHOM?

With the spring sun warming me through the French doors, I sat on the top step that led down to the laundry room, cell phone in hand. I was speaking to *him*, a classmate from long ago.

I leaned into the phone to hear better as he asked, "So what was your favorite country?"

"Oh, I don't know. They each had their own special flavor." *Flavor? We're not talking ice cream here.*

"Well, I once lived in Florida," he said, as if it were just around the corner and hardly worth mentioning.

"Florida's great. It's like a foreign country. Do you know how many alligators live there?"

"So if there are alligators, it makes a place, foreign?" he bantered.

As we chatted, the laughter flowed like water from our backyard pump that continued to run even after my three-year-old niece released the lever. I remembered how she held her hands under the water and giggled until it stopped.

That warm May afternoon, I let myself feel the laughter with the same abandon. Long after the call finished, I found myself smiling as some incidental comment came to mind.

May slipped into June and the calls increased until we spoke nearly every day. As we neared the end of June, I surprised him. "Guess what? My brother and I are headed to Toledo for the Fourth of July weekend. Do you live very far from there? If you can get there, I'm thinking, well…maybe, we can…."

He jumped in. "Meet? Or technically, meet again?"

I held my breath. Was a meet-up wise? Would the reality match up with what I had built in my mind?

He responded quickly. "Well, yeah. How could we not?"

I let out my breath, relief flooding through me. "We're just passing through, so we'll be in Toledo for a couple of hours."

"That's cool. There's a neat restaurant called Tony Packo's, if you want to meet there."

"Tony Packo's. That name sounds familiar…." It finally came to me. "That's from M*A*S*H. My family was a huge fan of that sitcom. Wasn't there some funny episode about Corporal Klinger radioing that restaurant for an order of some hot dogs?"

"That's the one. They were thirty-five-cent hot dogs. He convinced them to send them all the way to Korea during the war. That was a real restaurant in Toledo."

I laughed. "My brother's gonna love it. He's probably even been there. He watches all the re-runs. Yeah, that's a great idea!"

A short pause and the voice on the other end of the phone teased, "How will I know you?"

"I'll be the one with the cane."

"I'll wait for you in the parking lot," he said, "and lead you in."

"Are you out of your mind? I'll lead *you* in."

The next day, I received an email from him: *Who knows how these things happen? Funny how we started off chatting, sharing stories of each other's lives and the next thing you know, we're talking about meeting and who's going to lead the other into the restaurant when we're together.*

I barely saw the rest of the message. My eyes kept going back to those words. Who would be leading the other…a touchy subject.

I didn't learn to use my cane to have anyone *lead* me into any restaurant. Well, at least we were clear on that issue. I turned my attention to what I would wear on our date. Smart? Casual? Sophisticated? What outfit subtly radiated 'world traveler savvy?'

As I packed for our out-of-town trip, I jotted down a few essentials. *Toothbrush. Toothpaste. Cell phone charger. Oh yes, lipstick. Can't forget that.*

My brother and I rented a car for our trip to Ohio. He selected some old-fashioned, maroon car that looked like it came straight out of the fifties. We slapped my credit card on the table, and ten minutes later, we were on the road.

"It's a gorgeous afternoon," I said, watching the trees and gardens in full bloom pass by as we drove through town. All kinds of kids' outdoor gear—a little fuzzy—probably tricycles and lots of speed bikes, a wagon in one yard and a round blow-up pool in another whizzed past. It also seemed to be a day for washing cars. "Hey, what's going on there?" I asked as some blurry movement caught my eye.

"Where?"

"On the right."

My brother glanced my way and back to the road. He patiently described the scene. "Some kids are playing in the sprinkler."

"Oh, that's what it is."

That's the way it was for me. One minute things looked clear and the next, fuzzy. Movement sometimes caught me off guard because I couldn't hold a moving target in the "tunnel" part of my vision. Parts got cut off. It's like looking out of glasses with tri-focal lenses. Every tilt of your

112

head shifts the clarity.

I looked out the window again. Some houses owners hung American flags from their porches, others draped them. A few even spiked miniature versions in their yards. I loved seeing the patriotism surrounding the Fourth of July. All in all, it seemed like I was having a pretty good vision day.

On the throughway, I closed my eyes and leaned back against the seat, trying to imagine our upcoming reunion after more than thirty years.

"I can't wait to eat some of Tony Packo's hotdogs," my brother remarked. "I like the Hungarian sauce. It's kinda spicy."

"You going to get a T-shirt?"

"I might. I gotta see what they look like."

Who was he kidding? He collected them from all over. *I might just buy one for him. After all, he let me come with him.*

As afternoon merged into early evening, I felt my heart skip a few beats. What would my classmate—um, my *date*—think of me? I unzipped my purse and took out my lipstick. Other than needing to reapply that, my make-up was fine.

"Look for 280 on the Eastbound side," my brother said.

That made me smile. He'd see it long before a vision-impaired person would.

Soon we arrived. I took several deep breaths. I was sure my date would be waiting for us inside the restaurant. The excited flutter returned to my stomach.

At the door, I stopped. "Oh! I forgot my lipstick." I had put it in the dash while looking for the turn-off sign on the throughway. "If he's there, tell 'im I'll be right in. I need to go back and get my lipstick."

My brother reached for the door handle. "I'll probably recognize him from his picture. Don't take a long time."

I swept my cane ahead of me and crossed the road into the parking lot adjacent to the restaurant. Uh-oh. There were *four* identical parking lots, one on each corner of the four-way intersection. Which one did we park in? I would just have to check one by one. Great! I couldn't even see what color the cars were until I was right up on them. This would take longer than I thought.

"Maroon. His car is maroon," I muttered. It was slow-going. I peered inside all the car windows of the first parking lot, trying to figure out which one belonged to my brother, if any.

A woman materialized from out of nowhere. "May I help you?" She emphasized each word, like an old-fashioned schoolmarm, her implication clear. She might as well have accused me of checking out the goods in someone else's car.

"Um, I'm looking for...I mean, my brother's car is...I forgot something I need to take into the restaurant…you know, the famous one across the way. Just can't find…oh no, thanks, I'm okay. I don't need any help."

"Turn around and speak to me," the woman ordered. "You're too far away for me to hear. What are you holding?"

I slowly swung around, my cane tapping the blacktop in front of me.

The woman's expression wasn't clear at that distance. But she seemed to take a step back and that was probably due to my cane, which was in plain view.

How could I explain my peeking into car windows at sunset? What good upstanding person hung around parking lots doing that?

Retrieving a tube of coral lipstick sounded like one of my weak, fabricated stories. Funny how the truth sounded stranger than what anyone could dream up. As I saw it, I had two choices. Head back over to the restaurant and leave her with the impression I was doing something sneaky. That would also be admitting defeat. Or, tell her I needed something from my car and find something inside it more plausible than a tube of lipstick.

I knew when the light bulb went off in her head because her voice suddenly changed. "Are you…blind?"

That word grated on my nerves. "Well, yes and no. I can see close-up and…."

The woman put up her hand. "Wait here," she commanded, "I'll get help." Her voice brooked no argument.

So I waited, feeling foolish as the minutes ticked by. I wondered if my brother and my date had met and how they were getting along. Had they recognized each other? They were probably looking at a menu and wondering what had happened to me. I wanted to get inside the restaurant.

The sun was going down fast. It looked like a man was moving straight toward me from across the parking lot. He was! "You must be the girl. Are you lost?"

I didn't have to ask which girl. "Lost. No-o-o, not at all. I know where I am. It's the car that is lost."

The man assured me I didn't have to be afraid. "I'm an off-duty fireman," he explained, adding that he was a family man—a father and a husband.

Seriously? The lady hailed an off-duty fireman to rescue me? The kind that rescues lost dogs? It appeared he was now rescuing lost women from out of town.

"Thank you, but I'm perfectly capable of—"

"It's okay. It's okay. Name's Paul." He spoke kindly, using the same soft tone he might use to persuade a child to jump from a burning building—focused and intent.

I wanted to stomp my feet at his reassuring tone of voice. *I know that lady meant well but...I. Have. A. Cane.*

Be practical, I told myself. How many of the four parking lots would need to be searched before finding the right car? I sighed and pushed back my pride.

He's already here. I've been gone this long. At least he can help me find the car and retrieve my lipstick.

"I'm looking for a maroon vehicle. It's a rental car," I added, to head off questions about the make. Any other detail escaped my mind at that moment except for the generic, "It's big and clean."

"Let's see if we can find it. You want to take my arm?"

No. sir, I do not. You see this cane? I'm perfectly capable of walking on my own. "Thank you," I said, lightly taking the crook of his arm, finding it all around easier to give in.

As we crossed at the light, he slowed his pace to mine. "Your first time in Toledo? What brings you here?"

"Tony Packo's," I said, omitting the mention of my date.

"They pack a mean hotdog! Have you seen the signed buns?"

"Signed buns?"

"You'll find hundreds tacked to the walls. Celebrities come in and leave their signature on hotdog buns. Not only actors. Presidents sign 'em too. There's even one signed by an astronaut."

I warmed to this kind-hearted man who came—surely no questions asked—to help a blind woman find her rental car and a tube of lipstick stashed away in the dash. So much effort for a bit of vanity.

"Do you often rescue lost, blind women?"

"Wa-a-ll now, I've rescued a cat from the top of a tree. I've helped deliver a baby. And, of course, put out fires. But you're my first lost, blind woman."

"Hmm. At least you didn't have to climb up a ladder or tree to reach me."

The snicker that escaped his lips scored well with me. I felt more comfortable around him.

We found the car in the parking lot across the street. We hadn't even locked it. Once inside, I snatched my lipstick and slipped it into my purse. "Thanks for your help. If you could point me in the direction of the...."

"No, sirree. I couldn't do that." Why did I have to have a conscientious fireman who wouldn't let me cross the street alone? He took my hand in a fatherly way. I felt like a little kid. When we got to the door, I hesitated. How was I going to put my lipstick on in front of this man?

"Thank you," I said, hoping he'd get the message.

"I want to make sure you find your party," he replied, opening the heavy door and motioning for me to go in.

"Umm, well, I have my…okay." I didn't want to hurt his feelings.

He took my hand again.

I can't believe this just happened! After all the talk about who would be leading whom where, what could be worse than a real live off-duty fireman leading me into the restaurant? He might even think I planned this entrance as a joke.

Then I heard every woman's romantic dream greeting. "You…got…lost…in the parking lot?"

And who would have believed the first words out of my mouth would be a protest?

"The thing is, there were four *identical* parking lots and four identical crosswalks an'…."

"It's hard for her to see at night," my brother cut in helpfully. "She has to use a cane."

"I wasn't…*lost*…per se…." There went my she's-traveled-the-world-from-one-end-to-the-other reputation spiraling down. Not making it across the parking lot carried a lot more weight right then.

"Okay, I'll tell you about the adventure of how the off-duty fireman came to rescue me, but let's order first." As we ate our hotdogs loaded with the café's signature spicy Hungarian sauce, I regaled them with the whole story—well, not the whole story. I left out the lipstick part.

My brother wandered over to see the T-shirts and also to give us some time alone together. My late 'entrance' jumpstarted the conversation. The first 'blind' date awkwardness bypassed us.

The lipstick! "Um, I need to go to the restroom." I picked up my cane and stood up. Before my date could say a word, I rushed off to the powder room—which the waiter kindly pointed out to me—to apply my lipstick, fluff up my hair and freshen up. It must have taken me longer than I thought because I heard a tap on the door.

"Amy, are you…lost?"

I had led him to the restroom! If this was the start of a new relationship, I would definitely have to retrain his thinking in regard to my independence.

"Be right out." As I felt around for the hand blower or a paper towel dispenser—equipment always found in different locations—I narrowly escaped dipping my purse in the toilet as my cane fell sideways and hit the floor with a clatter.

"What's going on in there?" The second most coveted response a woman wants to hear from her date as she tries to muffle sounds in the bathroom. Flustered, I hurried out while plumping my coral-pink lips.

My date noticed the new color and whispered how beautiful I looked.

As he took my hand, my heart beat out a he-likes-me, he-likes-me refrain. We strolled around the restaurant, hand in hand, checking out the signed hotdog buns. We tried to find President Carter's and the astronaut's buns.

Then, just like that, it was time to leave. My brother went on ahead to give us time to say goodbye. We stood outside the restaurant making doe eyes at each other to delay the inevitable. My date latched onto my hand even more tightly. "You're not getting out of my sight—at least until we cross the parking lot," he whispered.

"My cane!"

"Huh?"

"It's in the bathroom. I left my *purse* there, too!" My purse had a ton of money I had withdrawn for the trip. I really needed to get that—pronto.

"Let me help you find it," he said, sounding a bit dazed at the quick turn of events.

"My purse?" I asked, still preoccupied with the money aspect of it.

"No. The restroom."

"Oh." Not a good plan. What man ever took his date to the restroom? I suddenly remembered the fireman. Huh, this time my *date* would be leading me! *This is a trick*, I thought, forgetting *I* was the one who forgot everything.

My date paid for our meal, and I didn't need to find my way around. For just a moment, I left my blindness behind as we moved forward holding hands, walking side by side, neither leading the other.

In the end, we compromised. The waiter helped me find the restroom. There, leaning against the wall, was my cane. I scanned the room for my purse. There it was, next to the toilet. Grabbing it, I checked my wallet for the cash. *Yep, all there.* I reapplied my lipstick before making my way back to the entrance, sweeping my cane ahead.

The compromise continued as we left the restaurant. I swept my cane forward with my right hand and held onto the crook of his arm with my left. This had nothing to do with need. It had everything to do with romance—on my terms.

Streetlights glared against the dark paved road. "The parking lot is across the street to the left," I said. As we paraded over, I heard three quick toots—a signal my brother and I had established to locate his car more easily—and paused.

My date walked me over to the passenger's side. There, he pulled me into a hug and kissed me goodnight. "I'll call you tomorrow," he whispered, as if he lived next door. "Don't get lost in any more parking lots tonight," he teased with a light smile and squeezed me tight. With a final kiss, he opened the door for me. "Got your cane. Your purse. Anything else?"

I shook my head, a little choked up.

He closed the door and walked around to the driver's side. The window came down and my date spoke. "Thanks for comin' tonight. Don't get too close to the fireworks and take care of your sister."

"You're welcome. We'll be back to Tony Packo's," my brother assured him and added, "She'll be okay. I'll watch out for her."

I had a feeling my life was going to take a turn for the better. We'd find ways to meet up. As my brother and I left the parking lot, we laughed about the funny events that had happened.

Sometimes this world traveler leads with a giant step forward over an ocean or desert. Sometimes she takes a step back to gauge how far she's come in a brand new country called Cane Confessions. The really good days are when she can find the medium between them both and choose which one to embrace.

24/ THE PHANTOM HUGGER

I love unplanned encounters. They create a feeling of belonging. Whether it's a stranger or someone I know, meeting up with someone unexpected cheers me up. That's why I'll never forget riding the subway in São Paulo, Brazil, where I met someone who lived four miles away from my hometown in the US.

Being close to home wasn't without its challenges though. One cold, blustery day, my friend, Susie, and I went to lunch at a Chinese restaurant in town. Afterward, we stopped at a nearby grocery store. We split up so we could each find what we needed. I made a quick circuit, picking up some frozen foods and a pound of ground beef, and checked out.

Waiting for Susie to finish up, I tucked myself into an out-of-the-way spot by the entrance. Blasts of cold air chilled me every time the door opened. I leaned on my cane with one hand and fished my cell phone out of my purse. One voice message. When I pressed the button to listen, it somehow switched to speaker phone.

"Meow," my friend said, instead of "hello." It was his way of making fun of me because he often says I let my cat call the shots with me.

Did anyone hear that? I quickly took it off speaker phone so I wouldn't draw any more attention. My cane did a good enough job of that by itself.

Some shoppers brushed by to check a shopping cart a few feet away; holiday goodies, from what little I could make out.

"They're half price. I'm gonna grab me a couple rolls," the first lady said. "Get a head start on next year."

Her companion muttered something, but she was walking away so I only heard the tail end of her response. "…You're a whore."

She was a *what?* I couldn't believe my ears! Had I heard her correctly? The first lady reached into the cart and pulled out a long package. I strained to see better, feeling like Gladys Kravitz, the nosy neighbor in the 60s sitcom, *Betwitched.* I craned my neck. She'd said something about getting rolls. Toilet paper? Paper towels? Ah, probably wrapping paper. Oh, a *hoarder*—that made more sense.

Their voices faded as they wandered further into the store.

Where are you, Susie? Hurry up.

A steady stream of shoppers passed by, slowing down slightly as our paths met. I stepped back, even more out of their way. I wore my old, ugly boots that day since the snow had turned to a slushy rain, making the parking lot a sopping mess. As I waited for Susie, I shuffled the worn and cracked vinyl heel of one boot in a pool of water that had gathered at my feet.

Something red and fuzzy lay on the floor a few inches away. I leaned down to get a closer look, but still couldn't tell what it was. Like a child who just *had* to find out, I bent over and touched it. *A glove.* Checking my coat pocket, I found one but not the other. *Ah, must have fallen out.* I was the Queen of Gloves, probably had the biggest motley collection in northwest Pennsylvania. When I picked up the glove, I found a muddy footprint on it. Someone had trampled it. I took a tissue from my purse and wiped it. Right then I noticed. This glove didn't match the one in my pocket. They were different shades of red and different thicknesses. I dropped it quickly and giggled at myself. *Let me make that the Queen of Unmatched Gloves.*

"Mommy, what's that lady holding?"

I glanced up to find a child tugging at his mother's pant leg and pointing at my cane as they passed by. I quickly folded my cane in half and put it out of sight.

A blurry form slowed down, but instead of moving past me like the other shoppers, it stopped next to me. "Amy, how ya' doin'?" The body leaned in and gave me a hug.

I hugged him back as if I knew exactly who he was. It was so fast, the only clue I could grasp was that I came up to his shoulders.

Who is this Phantom Hugger?

This was no ordinary, 'sorry bud, how do I know you?' situation. This was RP playing tricks on my eyes again—big time. Every once in a while, my vision blurred so much I couldn't recognize people. It was happening more frequently in my vision-loss journey. I needed details—eye color, nose type, cheeks, chin, hair color and style—all these things would help me discern who I was speaking to. All I had to go on was blur.

So, focus on the voice.

The voice sounded deep, kind of playful, like someone I should know—but who?

My sleuthing skills kicked in. It was a man's voice—someone who knew me, well enough to give me a hug. Taller than me. He probably lived right here in my hometown. Good strong clues here.

"I'm doing great. How was your Christmas?" I asked.

"Aah, y'know."

No clue there. "Yeah. What did Santa bring ya'?"

"Santa didn't visit this year," he confided, "but I did receive a brand new hopper to brew beer. I'm lookin' forward to trying it out."

Do I know anyone who brews beer? Could he be a relative? How do I know *that voice?*

Back to the investigation. "Wow, who gave that to you?" I half expected him to say he bought it for himself since Santa didn't come to his house.

He sounded startled. Did he think I was being nosy? "My girlfriend, Cecie."

"Oh-h." Cecie? Didn't ring a bell. *He's definitely not a relative. I know all their girlfriends.*

"He received a grill, too."

Wait a minute. Who said that? My head whipped around as I tried to pinpoint a new voice. A man's body materialized. *Did he suddenly arrive or has he been standing there the whole time?* The second figure was a tall, husky guy with a long, long beard.

I kind of wanted to laugh. Here was this big, tall guy whose most obvious feature was a long beard. This dude showed up out of nowhere. Like...Santa Claus! Coincidental? Christmas was last week. *Ah, this RP drives me crazy. Should I hug him too? Should I wait for him to hug me?*

I normally enjoyed running into people—but not like this. *Just keep smiling. Make eye contact. That blobby thing is his face. Look toward the top. Does he have hair? Oh my, I don't think he does. Good clue!*

I mentally scrolled down the list of people I knew and who my friends knew that would recognize me. Two people. Friends of friends? I drew a blank. Who did I know who didn't have hair? Who had a long beard? Who could they be?

I heard a woman's voice as she strode toward us. *Could this be Cecie?* "Sorry to interrupt, but do either of you two men know the best kind of kindling to buy for a fireplace?"

Not Cecie. She wouldn't have addressed them that way. No, probably a stranger. I bristled. *Why did she only ask the men? Why did she assume I didn't know anything about firewood?* In fact, I did. My father and brother were tree fellers. So I knew a little something about kindling.

As the conversation continued, and I was ignored, it gave me time to figure out what was going on. The newcomer was flirting with the Phantom Hugger and Bearded Man. I bet she wasn't even interested in buying any kindling.

Just as I expected, she walked right past the small bundles of kindling for sale stacked against the wall. *Great. I see the starter wood but not the people I'm talking to.* I'd often heard RP was like being able to see an elephant on the other side of the room but tripping over the pencil at your feet. That day I really understood that expression.

Frankly, I was glad when she left so I could continue my investigation. Clearing my throat and trying to get back on track, I shivered when another cold gust of air hit me as a new shopper entered the store. "Sure is chilly out there."

"Come on, wimp," he teased. "This weather is nothing like Alaskan winters."

My ears pricked up. *Alaska? Okay, now we're getting somewhere.*

I took a guess. "You lived in Alaska, not just visited, right?"

"Darn tootin' I did. Thirty-five years." He sounded proud. I guess I would be proud, too, if I ever stayed in one place long enough. "Talk about sub-zero temps and wind chill. Heck, you can't even get in or out most of the time unless you fly in."

Bingo! My brain worked out what the obstacle was and overcame it, like a mental mobility cane.

The Phantom Hugger had to be Brian, one of my high school classmates. I hadn't seen him since our high school reunion the year before. "I'm so glad you stayed in the area," I enthused. "Although I don't know why you'd ever choose Pennsylvania over Alaska. Have you seen the Northern lights? Ah, the wildlife alone...." *Now,* we had something to talk about.

I was ready to jump in and have a real conversation when my classmate said, "We'd better get going now. Great seein' ya'."

Wish I could say the same.

Shortly after the two men left, Susie finished her shopping. Strangely enough, my vision returned. My moments of confusion were over.

I set my groceries in her cart and pulled my hat down to cover any limp and flattened hair. That was also my ugly hat day. On the way to the parking lot, I filled Susie in on the chance meeting.

"Why didn't you just say, 'Who are you?'"

"Hark, who goes there?" I shouted in my best Shakespearean voice.

"No seriously, why didn't you say you didn't recognize him? It's so much easier than playing twenty questions."

The tip of my cane slid in the slush, and I caught it to avoid a fall. When we reached her vehicle, I said, "It might be easier, but not nearly as fun."

She opened her car door, slid in and turned on the ignition. "What's the real problem?"

I sighed. "I just can't do it. I know it sounds easy to say, 'Sorry, I'm having a bad vision day. I can't see you. So *who* are you?' It feels...somehow embarrassing...to admit I don't know who I'm talking to."

"So you'd rather pretend?"

"Well, in a way, yes." I tried to explain. "It's difficult when people don't identify themselves, especially if I've only seen someone once in thirty-five years." I shook my head. "Half the time, people don't even notice my cane, even when it's out in the open and I'm just standing."

Susie shifted into reverse and backed out of the space. She looked confused. "Didn't you say the other day it bothered you when people stared?"

"Both things happen." I sighed again. "Maybe I can assign a secret code to everyone and make them say it before I speak to them."

"That'll be fun for you to keep on top of the zillion other passwords you keep losing."

I smiled. "I think I'll just move to Alaska. Fly myself in during the start of winter. It's so remote, I'll never meet up with anyone I don't know. That'll solve my problem. You see how practical I am?"

"Good one, Amy. Only you hate the cold."

Susie was right—about a lot of things. I would have to come to terms with being out in public and find a smoother way to handle the situation. After all, I didn't plan to barricade myself indoors. With my vision growing progressively worse, bumping into family and friends would happen more often and I'd probably have more trouble recognizing people.

About a year earlier, I experienced the opposite—where an older church member didn't seem to recognize *me* at all. When I saw Laura, I gave her a hug. She introduced herself and said, "We're so glad to see you here."

I took a step backward. Did she think I was a *visitor?* Didn't she *recognize* me? She knew me well. We had even served food at the City Mission together for over six months. As soon as I could, I escaped to a pew and buried myself in the bulletin, re-reading the announcements. I wanted to blurt out, "It's me, Amy. I'm a regular member. I grew up in this church."

Sometime later, I read an article posted to one of my sight support groups. It focused on social etiquette to help sighted people know how to interact with people who are blind. It mentioned the importance of identifying oneself since the vision-impaired person might not recognize or remember someone by voice alone.

Ahh. That made sense. Laura had introduced herself to me *only* after I opened up about my vision loss to the church. She had done her homework. At the time, I easily recognized her, but she didn't know how much I could see. She probably wanted to help me as much as possible. Instead, it only made me think she'd become forgetful. Now I understood and appreciated the gesture.

That night, I compared the incident from both angles. While my classmate was the Phantom Hugger in the store, I was the Phantom Hugger at church. I giggled at the latter. In each situation, I served as the silent partner in not responding to the needs of the situation. Instead, I only reacted in survival mode. I learned I need to take the initiative. When I think back to how Laura took time to make sure I knew who she was, these days I'm encouraged to do my part. Maybe next time I'd be more assertive.

Meanwhile, when I talked to my classmate again, he said, "You had me totally fooled, Amy. I really had no idea you didn't recognize me right from the start. You looked like you were making eye contact." I'm just proud enough to take that as a compliment. Oh, and the man with the beard? Not Santa. It was Brian's brother and he was there all along.

It's good to see the humor even when you can't see the person.

25/ BUDDY TO THE RESCUE

Thick frost on the windowpane nearly obscured the snow steadily falling on that January morning. Itching for change, I forced myself to take a walk in the fresh air. Just the type of day my beautiful black Lab had relished. Bundled in coat and gloves, I felt a pang in my gut as I passed the snowbank—I called it 'the Fort.' Buddy used to burrow through tunnels he made, popping up now and again with a big, goofy grin on his face to see if I was watching. Who would ever dream a dog born in the Middle East would love winter so much? November, December, January. Three months now since he'd crossed over the Rainbow Bridge. Brushing the tears away, I returned home.

Inside, I settled at my computer with a cup of hot cocoa and checked my phone messages. Someone by the name of Heather Smart had called. She was in charge of Leader Dogs for the Blind and was a member of the Lions Club. She wanted me to be a speaker for some event.

Yes!

I hit the call back button and waited for Heather to pick up. She asked me if I were interested in being the featured speaker for their Dinner in the Dark fundraiser.

She wants me not just to speak but be the featured speaker! It took me a moment to digest that news.

"Our event focuses on both the blind *and* their leader dogs," Heather explained. "The highlight is a fancy, sit-down meal. The caveat is that the guests can't see what they're eating since they're wearing sleep shades. This is to help bring awareness to how people who are blind go through every day. That's where the name, 'Dinner in the Dark,' comes from."

"Yeah, that makes sense. What's a leader dog?"

"It's another name for a guide dog. Most of the speakers will focus on that topic, and the money raised will go to a long overdue, completely revamped leader dog facility in Michigan."

"I was just missing my dog," I said quietly. "I think this is the perfect opportunity to honor him. He wasn't a guide dog—just a wonderful rescue animal." Disappointment washed over me. She probably had me confused with someone else. "Hang on, why do you want me? Um, I've never owned a leader dog or any dog for the blind."

"That's the thing," Heather sounded excited. "We want you to talk about your mobility journey—that is, with your cane. Good cane skills are a must before any candidate trains with a companion dog."

"Oh-h. Okay." I brightened, taking a sip of cocoa. "In that case, I accept. Only one other question: how did you find out about me?"

"Your book trailer. It made me cry. Your story matches up perfectly with our goals. We'll have you talk about coming to terms with your vision loss and what you did in your mobility training. Then follow it up with how leader dogs impact a person's life. I'm so happy you've agreed to be our speaker. I love you already."

The trailer. Another blogger had helped me find the perfect song to complement the slide show I put together of me using my white cane. The song highlighted my faith journey as I learned to embrace a different way of "seeing."

Seated at my desk, holding onto my half-full cup of cocoa, I glanced out the window. Gusts of snow blew through the street, creating snow drifts on the other side. Likewise, I felt a wave of happiness sweep through me, creating warm drifts on the inside.

Heather's words tumbled out, one after the other. "I can't wait to know you better. You're even a dog lover. How would you like to join our planning committee? We meet every couple of weeks over dinner. Do you like Italian food? Come on, you know you want to."

I wasn't sure how often speakers joined in on the planning of an event, but I thought it would be a great opportunity to get to know more about the Lions Club.

When I arrived, they treated me like a celebrity author—shaking my hand, asking me about my book and making me feel at home in their midst. The committee members came from different Lions Clubs around the district, so meeting them enabled me to glimpse what the Lions Club was like on a wider scale.

As our planning meeting progressed, they often asked my opinion on the dinner from a vision-impaired perspective. For example, "What kinds of information should our coaches tell the diners when they first come to the table?"

"Well, by then, they'll be wearing sleep shades, right? They'll need to have an idea where their table setting is in relation to them. It would be good for table coaches to familiarize them with it by using time coordinates. For example: 'Your silverware is at three. Your glass is at one, etc.' Same with the food on the plate."

Later they asked me if the table coach should reassure the diners that, if they felt stressed, they could take off their sleep shades.

"I don't think that's a good idea," I warned. "I can't change my way of seeing when I feel stressed. Let the diners experience some anxiety. They might peek, but, no, don't give them permission to remove them. It'll undermine what the dinner is trying to accomplish."

By seeking my opinion, they gave me an important role in helping to plan the event. In fact, they helped me find my voice. It didn't happen all at once, but over the next couple of months, I started volunteering some of my own ideas.

One Saturday evening, my cell phone rang. "Amy, Heather here. The meeting will be at the Riverside Inn tomorrow. You comin'? I'll pick ya' up around eleven," she said without giving me time to refuse.

I should be writing these dates on my calendar. "I…guess so."

When I heard the car beep the next afternoon, I ran down the steps from my apartment and hopped into the car so fast I didn't even open my cane.

Heather's hand was still sitting on the horn as if she hadn't had time to remove it. "How did you do that?"

"Do what? Oh, you mean, get here so fast?"

"No, get here without your cane?"

"This is home—familiar territory. Plus, it's a sunny day." Better be careful. I might appear so skillful she might say, "Keep on runnin' girl, right past the gig. Only slow-walkin' blind people need apply." I smiled. Too late for that.

In the car, Heather explained why we needed to drive forty-five minutes to Cambridge Springs for the meeting. "Believe me, there's a purpose. The committee needs to see what the Riverside Inn is like, taste-test their food and finalize the menu. You can get a feel for where you'll be speaking and selling your books."

"Sure, that will be helpful."

"Have you ever been there? It's a Victorian-era inn, antique furniture and what have you. You're going to absolutely love it when you see it," she enthused, not even realizing what she'd just said.

Ahh, what I see remains…to be seen. Hopefully, it'll stay a good vision day.

When we arrived, I unfolded my cane and climbed the steps onto the smooth planks of the hundred-year-old porch with ease, enjoying the nice breeze.

"You do fantastic with your cane," Heather commented. "I didn't even have to tell you where the steps were."

"Canes have step sensors," I said with a straight face. "Kind of like those machines that beep when they come across money." She wasn't going to buy that. "Nah, I can see better on a sunny day."

But once inside, I slowed way down. *That's what you get for acting so cocky.* The interior was like a maze. Hard to see anything in the dim lighting. The furniture had claw-like feet that kept catching on my cane. *I hate this furniture. It's clunky and crowded.* It was difficult to tell where one room ended and another began.

Stephanie—at least that's who I thought it was in the murky light—

called out, "Are you okay, Amy?"

"Sure," I said, just before nearly toppling over a floor lamp, which emitted the smallest halo of light I had ever seen.

She reached out a hand to steady me. "Would you like to take my arm?"

"I think so." I reached for her elbow at the same time I stubbed my toe. "Aaah!"

"Are you all right?" She sounded concerned.

I gulped. "Never better." I tried to sound more cheerful than I felt.

At last, seated at a spacious, lacquered, probably oak table, I relaxed and folded up my cane.

"You're safe now," Stephanie said, taking a seat next to me. "Feel better?"

"All I have to say is this is the perfect venue to challenge your diners in sleep shades, if they don't kill themselves beforehand," I said in a low voice only she could hear.

"Oh, they won't put on the sleep shades until right before they're taken to their tables," she said quickly.

"Good thing."

The committee members hashed out various courses and prices for the dinner while the waitress delivered our beverages. She set a goblet of water in front of me.

I stared at the glass. Clear, heavy glasses were the worst to deal with. Transparent meant I couldn't always distinguish the inside from the outside of the glass, and feeling for it led to dumping it over. The heavier it was, the harder it crashed. I wavered between wanting to glug the water down and sipping it to be polite. The best compromise was to handle it as little as possible. I thought about pointing the glass issue out to the committee, but figured that if the diners used them, they would probably get a better idea of vision challenges, so I remained silent.

We stopped talking long enough to order lunch.

When I heard the final menu included gravy and a tossed salad, I spoke up. "I wonder how diners will distinguish the gravy from the salad dressing? That should make for some interesting conversation." I chuckled.

"Really? You think that will cause a problem?"

"Hmm, it could." I swirled the ice carefully in my water goblet. "Especially if they're served in similar containers."

Before we could launch into a new topic, the waitress said, "There's one more choice you need to make. Which butter would you like served with our specialty breads? You can taste them yourselves to decide."

She arrived shortly with the samples: slices of cranberry and nut breads wrapped in a cloth napkin. The bread basket included three small silver dishes, each containing a round, flavored ball of whipped butter: plain, maple and cinnamon.

"Anyone have a preference?" one Lion club member asked.

"How 'bout this? We take all three," I said, excitedly. "Look, they all come in identical containers, so the guests can get a surprise burst of flavor on their bread. It'll make it more fun."

"I like that," Heather said. "I think you're onto something there."

It was the last meeting, and I'd learned a lot, not only about speaking up, but also how dedicated these committee members were, in particular to serving those with vision loss. Some also worked with leader dogs. Every time we met, I thought of Buddy.

On one occasion, I told a story about Buddy's devotion. Heather said, "Do you want a leader dog? We can help you get one."

I thought for a moment. "No, I don't think so." The timing wasn't right. I had responsibilities at home that prevented me from taking the month-long training. "Definitely later." Besides, at that moment I didn't think any dog could replace Buddy, even a leader dog who would help me see.

The morning of the speaking engagement, I had my make-up done by a professional beautician in town. "Your eyes are your best feature," she said. "This will make them pop." She carefully outlined each eye with a dark brown pencil.

The comment about my eyes made me chuckle—more like my biggest flaw, I'd say. And the thought of them 'popping' during my talk made me think of firecrackers going off. But it was uncanny that my being in a position to bless others came about only as a result of the weaknesses in my eyes. Our God delights in turning the tables.

I wore a sparkling black, sleeveless shift and a short, fashionable, white jacket for the evening. With my eye-popping make-up and my new clothing, I felt gorgeous. However, my stomach was doing flip-flops as I mentally rehearsed my talk.

First, I had to get through dinner. We all had to get through dinner.

Each table coach in turn held up a sign with a large number printed on it. In case anyone missed the sign, an announcer called the table number over the intercom as well. The diners had received a notice in the mail beforehand with their assigned table numbers. Mine was the last, so I watched the earlier groups line up, all wearing sleep shades and holding onto the shoulder of the one in front—like kindergarteners. The line looked hilarious.

But the diners listened and followed directions, shuffling off to their respective tables with nervous laughter. I never saw anyone let go until he or she sat down at the table. It seemed kind of silly for me to wear sleep shades, but I finally put them on too. Since I was the featured speaker, I didn't want to be a rebel.

After the meal, Heather played my book trailer. There was a problem with the sound and it didn't come on until halfway through the song. *That's what I get for being first.* I used my cane and walked confidently to the center of the room. As the song drew to a close, I tried to calm my nerves.

It was Buddy who came to the rescue. "The day I was invited to speak to your group, I was missing my dog terribly," I ad-libbed. "Then this bright and cheerful voice came over the phone line and said, 'We want you to speak at our fundraiser, one that highlights dogs.' I felt like Buddy was right there, pushing me with his snout to move ahead and stop mourning him. So I'm here today because of a cold nose and a warm heart, just like all of you are…."

I told them my story, gaining courage and confidence as I went.

When I finished, Heather, teary-eyed, hugged me. "Your talk was awesome! Now go and sell your books."

A few weeks later, when the stardom dimmed, I was invited to join a recently-formed Lions Club in our county. Stephanie, a lifetime Lion—a member whose parents and grandparents also served as members—emphasized the benefits of joining the group. "Since it's brand new, you can help shape it. They need you," she said. "As you discovered, vision loss is a big outreach within the Lions Club community. Having you in the club will be a strong reminder of why we do what we do."

"What exactly do you do?"

"We serve."

I remembered that snowy day in January, itching for some kind of change in my life. I recalled seeing the wind sweep the snow over the road and immediately after, feeling happiness sweep through me. It was the wind of positive change, and amazingly, my cane and mobility training was at the center of it. I fought the idea of a cane for so long, and yet look what came out of it—independence, increased confidence and a club I could help shape.

"I would like to join the West County Lions Club," I said quietly. "I'm an encourager. But I'm not sure about this 'serving' business. I used to be a waitress and dumped a tray carrying eight glasses of ice water onto a table full of patrons. The baby and the grandpa howled—and neither of them got wet!"

When she laughed, I said, "Are you sure you want me?"

"We'll take you, but we'll leave the ice water to someone else."

The financial commitment concerned me too, but Stephanie said, "Each member's financial status varies. What one can't pay, another does. At the heart of the Lions Club is our service."

Reassured, I made my commitment. A year later, I was sworn in as secretary—another comical example of God's delight in turning the tables.

26/ MT. FUJI: MOVE HIGH THE STONES

As spring turned to summer, the talk among my Japanese students at the American Navy base revolved around climbing Mount Fuji in July and August. They assumed all their teachers would jump—rather, climb—at the opportunity.

Suzuki-san said, "We have special saying: 'A wise man climb Fuji-san once; a fool climb twice.'"

That piqued my curiosity. "Why is he a fool to climb it twice?"

"Ve-ly high." He gestured with his hands. "Take too much time."

Students then hashed over how high, a spirited conversation that shot back to Japanese. Someone looked it up. "It's 3,776 meters," he reported.

"So what is that in feet?" I asked.

Again, a flurry of words—in broken English and Japanese. Yoshida-san, my quietest student, took out his calculator and ended the discussion. "Miss Amy, 12,388 feet."

I couldn't miss out on this challenge! My supervisor, Frank, and his wife, Pat, were planning a night climb in mid-August, during the height of the climbing season. No other teachers seemed interested. My heart sank. A night climb for someone with night blindness and poor peripheral vision didn't seem wise, even once.

I asked questions, researched and schemed ways to adapt to the task. Finally, I decided to go with Frank and Pat. Mount Fuji was divided into ten stations. They planned to drive to the base of the mountain, park the van and walk to the fifth station, which was the starting point. We would take the Gotemba Trail, the lowest of four trails, to the tenth station—the summit.

The students egged me on in my pursuit to climb.

"You can to buy a climbing sticky. It help you move high the stones. Many sellers burn for memory." For a small fee, climbers could have the stick they bought engraved with the number of each station in Kanji as a souvenir. That sounded like my kind of adventure. I definitely wanted an engraved sticky.

"You can go far, teacher?" one student asked. "I think you must to prepare."

I heeded the advice. To prepare myself, I trekked up the steep winding pathways to Shinto shrines—the highest elevations in any Japanese city. Even then, after several attempts I couldn't make it up to the shrine without slowing to a very slow pace. But after four or five tries, I began to develop some muscles and that gave me confidence.

On the night of the big climb I put on two pairs of blue jeans, socks, sturdy sneakers, a T-shirt, sweatshirt, jacket and warm hat even though it was August. The wind speed at that height could blow up to fifty miles per hour. I also found a mining light to wear on my head for extra lighting. I couldn't forget food, some yen to buy *soba*—buckwheat noodles climbers traditionally slurp up before the climb—and the walking stick to aid me in my journey.

Soon we left for Hakone prefecture, where my adventure began. At 6:30 in the evening, we arrived at the fifth station. My heart beat erratically as I faced the challenge before me. *I can do this!*

In the beginning, the climb seemed too easy. I didn't even need my stick. Bright lights shone on the pathway. Hordes of people milled around. Laughter abounded. Friends chatted. Old people jogged past. My companions and I chatted as we wound our way around the broad slope together.

But not for long.

It became more challenging. Gradually, Frank moved ahead. Concerned for me, Pat adjusted herself to my slower pace. Since I had to watch the ground so carefully, I urged her ahead. "I've got my light. Don't worry." I waved her away, downplaying my vision challenges. "Go catch up with Frank. I'll be fine."

The more intense concentration tired me out as the climb grew steeper. Finally, I rested.

I'm so slow and clumsy. Everyone is passing me up. If I could only see better, I'd be like everyone else. But I can do this. I can!

About midnight, I became less certain.

The pathway narrowed. Volcanic rock stood out like boulders, looming ahead. My light served little use. With one hand, I grasped onto volcanic sediment and bare roots, pulling myself up. With my other hand, I clutched my walking stick.

With so much necessary strong concentration, I didn't see the *ooji-san*, a little old Japanese man with a white goatee, pass me. "*Gambatte kudasai!*" he called out, "Do your best!" He waved his baseball cap before striding off full of bounce.

That hour several older Japanese climbers swung past me, joking and laughing. "*Gambatte kudasai,*" they all encouraged. I smiled, buoyed by their support.

As I continued my solitary ascent, Mount Fuji's picture-perfect, snow-capped image faded. Up close it looked ugly—barren volcanic rubble littered with rubbish.

In the wee hours of the morning, something scary happened. Someone pushed me and I fell down between two boulders. I lay there a few minutes before attempting to move. No one even noticed I'd fallen. Shocked, tears welled up in my eyes. I threw up a quick prayer. As I wiggled free from the two rocks, an older Japanese climber—a woman—reached out a hand and gently tugged me to my feet before going on her way.

Right around the curve, the path narrowed and a number of climbers bottlenecked. Craning my neck, I tried to see what the hold-up was. Surprisingly, I found myself stuck in the middle of a traffic jam on the mountain in the early morning shadows. We all inched forward in unison like ants on a stick. It dawned on me that, by being tightly sandwiched between climbers, the danger of my falling had decreased dramatically.

I continued pacing myself. The altitude made me light-headed and I stopped briefly, fearing another fall if I got too dizzy. My breath came in ragged gasps in the higher atmosphere. *Just keep going. Put one foot in front of the other.*

By that time, I had passed the sixth, seventh and eighth stations. At each station, I stood in line to get my climbing stick engraved. At the eighth, I purchased some steaming *udon* and sank to the ground, slurping it up from the Styrofoam bowl with the cheap, wooden chopsticks. Then I downed the leftover broth. Like the gentle tide coming in from the sea, a wave of warmth coursed through me. My nose constantly dripped from the colder temperatures, and I used my last napkin to wipe it before tossing that too into the Styrofoam bowl and then both into a steel-woven trash bin.

I rested on my haunches like my Japanese counterparts, taking swigs of bottled water and rubbing my thinly-gloved hands together to generate warmth. Thank God for the gloves that came with my climbing stick. I'd forgotten to bring my own.

I reluctantly stood up to continue the trek to the ninth station. The wind blew through me and I pulled my cap down to cover my ears.

This calls for a cup of green tea before I start again. One look at the line changed my mind. *No way I'm waiting for that line. I have a sunrise to meet!*

The ninth station came into view at around five-thirty. *Almost to the top. Almost. Keep going. Come on, lift up those legs! Move it! Go-temba! Go, Amy!* As I climbed the trail, I cheered my body on, wondering whether Frank and Pat had already made it and were waiting to see the sunrise.

The high altitude made me nauseous again and slowed me down. Thank goodness I had climbed up the pathways to the Shinto shrines. That preparation gave me some stamina so I could keep moving. I expelled a breath of air and rubbed the temples of my head. Someone offered me a few slices of lemon. I called out to the retreating figure, "*Domo! Domo!*" A slight bow. Then I popped a slice into my mouth and grimaced at the sour taste. *"Wa-wa-wa!"* Licking my chapped lips, I chewed on the skin before spitting it out. Grabbing a few crackers, I rested for a moment. *Let's go! Come on! Get back on the trail!*

By that point, I didn't care if I saw the once-in-a-lifetime Fuji-san sunrise. In fact, I didn't care if I took another step. Could I make it to the top? I lifted myself up with the stick, and let out a long breath. *I only need one more engraving to make this sticky complete. I can do it.* I blew a kiss to my stick and leaned on it to help me up.

The majestic peak of Mount Fuji finally emerged from cloudy vapor. I crumpled my flag into a ball, touching the ground with the fiery red circle of Japan's emblem and then pressing it to my heart before tying it back on the walking stick. It seemed fitting. I had reached the tenth station! At 12,388 feet, the wind nearly blew me down.

As the sun rose higher, I shed my mining light and layers of extra clothing. Daylight brought new confidence to my steps. But it also made me aware of how badly I needed a bathroom break. To top it off, I had no idea where my companions were.

"Ohayo-gozaimasu!" called a male climber who looked to be about twenty-five.

"G'morning!"

"I can see you have trouble going down. I help. Make your legs like this," he instructed, bowing the bottoms of his legs inward. "It make you strong grip. So you can't to fall on rocks."

"Do-mo," I said, elongating the 'o' as I thanked him.

Finding a captive audience, he continued talking as he fell into step with me.

"You vely tired. You no folget put the legs like this," he reminded, as I lurched amid an avalanche of small rubble.

My ankles were starting to weaken, refusing to adequately support my feet.

"When I no feer happy, I sing. You know Loberta Frack?" He launched into one of her songs—in excellent English. Both his l's and r's came out properly.

After adopting me, my guardian kept up the constant banter and singing, which made me feel cross, in light of my current struggles.

"I really need a toilet!" I moaned. "Where can I go?"

"Oh, I see. Toiret big ploblem now." He scanned the area before giving me his rendition of the current hit, "YMCA," with hand gestures.

I wanted to strangle him.

When it seemed that I couldn't wait a moment longer, my friend pointed out a tiny shack. Exhausted, I crossed over to it, stumbling into other climbers—mostly Japanese—who, with surprisingly good grace, caught me before I toppled us both over. As my energy decreased, so did my vision. My ankles trembled. In the shack, I finally, finally, found relief after hours of waiting.

With that problem behind me, I smiled at my companion and we continued on our way.

At ten o'clock that morning, we reached our starting point, the fifth station. "Big shame. I go my home now." He didn't seem to want to leave me until I met my friends. "You wait me. No move." He returned a few minutes later. "Come now," he pulled my arm. "We find Amy-san's boss."

He took me to a tag board covered with messages. I despaired of finding one for me. But I did. "Amy-san! *Don't* move from this spot!" Frank had signed it. My friend cheered. "You find rettel!"

Retell? Oh, letter. Yes, I had found the letter I needed.

Frank and Pat found me chatting in Japanese with my escort. I waved my walking stick with the Japanese flag and gloves tied to it. What a cool souvenir with the wood stamps! It represented all the adventure of the climb in six neat engravings.

Half an hour later, I steeped in the steaming, muddied *ofuro,* massaging my bruised and tender muscles in Hakone, an area famous for its hot springs. I recalled my laughter, fears, frustrations and the encouraging locals I met along the way.

Equipped with a lone mining light, shining far enough ahead for me to see where to place my feet, I had somehow found my way up Fuji-san through the mostly-dark climb. Who would have ever believed a woman with night blindness could climb the highest mountain in Japan? It was faith and the climbing sticky that helped me continue. That piece of wood with its brown Kanji engravings symbolized the adventure of the experience for me.

Years later, I see that uniquely-engraved walking stick as a crude forerunner to my cane. When I was walking the broad path at the bottom of the Gotemba Trail leading up Fuji-san, using the walking stick seemed unnecessary. But as I got to the huge volcanic boulders higher up, I started to depend on my walking stick.

The journey with my mobility cane parallels that of my walking stick. At first I didn't want it—certainly didn't need it. Unlike the Fuji-san walking stick, there was no adventure in having a cane. When my trainer first handed it to me, it came with a mental stamp emblazoned on it: BLIND. But that was short-lived. I needed to view my cane in the same perspective as I did my walking stick, embracing the adventure of where it took me, along with its usefulness. Each dent engraved on the cane reminds me I'm still moving forward. I haven't given up.

I did climb Fuji-san twice, so I could be viewed as a fool according to the Japanese proverb. The first time was to see if I could do it. The second time was to savor the experience.

Now, as a vision-impaired person, I conquer new mountains every day and cheer myself on, *"Gambatte kudasai!"*

27/ GETTING MY FEET WET AGAIN

It had been ten years since I'd traveled anywhere outside the United States. I had even allowed my passport to expire.

Bobbie, my high school classmate, and her husband were taking their first cruise with some friends to the Bahamas. When she found out I was losing my vision, she asked her husband if she could, as a surprise, invite me along as their guest. He agreed. She discussed options with the travel agent and learned if I didn't mind staying in the same room, the cruise line would provide us with a pull-down bed and I could travel at a reduced fare. I was indeed thrilled and surprised by her generous invitation.

Aside from a short trip from Cairo to Upper Egypt years earlier, I had never taken a cruise. It might be just the thing for me. Not only was I touched by her offer, I really did need a break at that point and had never traveled to the Caribbean. This would be a wonderful shared experience for us. A cruise would also be a great way to test how independent I could be with my cane.

But after talking it over with my family, I wasn't sure if it would work out. Three of us live together at home—my mom, my older brother and me. Mom kept us on a schedule, my brother drove us to appointments and I cooked dinner, split the chores with Mom and kept her company. It worked out well.

How could I leave for ten days?

"I think you should go," my brother said. "I would."

Mom hesitated, then nodded. "We can work something out."

I didn't feel comfortable leaving my family to cope with meals on their own, since cooking was too much for Mom to take on. But my nieces promised to help out by bringing food regularly. I set up a meal and visiting schedule for every day I would be gone. With a team of volunteers in place, I felt ready to go.

I phoned my friend. "Well, yeah, that sounds great. I'd love to go. We have a plan in place here," I told her.

"I'm so glad," Bobbie said, "Now's the time to go when you still have some vision left."

I agreed. I certainly didn't want to pass up the opportunity.

My new passport came. I turned the pages, wondering what kind of visas and stamps would fill them—and what kind of memories.

The day for our departure finally came. Bobbie, her husband, Jamie, and I drove to New York City to board the Norwegian Gem the following day.

The boarding area looked similar to an airline terminal. We had sent the suitcases on ahead, so I had only my purse and cane to worry about.

The intake process went quickly, and we each received a yellow plastic key card, which also served as the method of payment for everything on the cruise.

After the ship pulled out of the harbor, it seemed all the passengers headed directly to the top deck to wave goodbye to the city that never sleeps and the Statue of Liberty. A sharp wind whipped through my light T-shirt. I had to brace myself to take a picture of the majestic figure on Ellis Island. I couldn't stay long. The wind was brisk...and cold. Our cabin, Room 9106, was easy to find from the elevator. A left and another left.

Every floor had signs at the elevator. "We need to get oriented," I said, trying to create a mental map of the ship's floor plan. "Where is everything located?"

As Jamie read the list aloud, I studied it, trying to memorize which floors had buffets and restaurants, where to go for sports, the pool and observation decks. I noted the shows were on the ninth deck and the music lounges on the eighth. Two flights of carpeted stairs led up to the next deck or down to the preceding deck.

I wanted to get a feel for where things were so I could move around independently and give my friends time to be on their own. It seemed easy enough.

Early the next morning, I slipped into the bathroom to dress. Back in the room, I tiptoed so as not to wake my shipmates. The theme song to *The Pink Panther* ran through my head. Maybe because I was so smooth under cover. I grabbed my cell phone, which would calculate my steps, and located my cane. Quietly...I was out the door.

When I tried to close it, the door hit some mysterious soft obstruction. I pushed harder...it met with the same resistance. Then it swung open. Two seconds later, the mystery was solved. In the dim light, I discovered it was a man's leg. Jamie's leg.

He was standing right behind me, but hadn't been quick enough to slip through the door in time. As I was walking to the door, he must have jumped from the drop-down bed and slipped in behind me. Or else I'd walked right past him. He was standing in the doorway.

Jamie had been even more covert than me.

My face felt hot. "Oh, Jamie, I didn't know you were awake. I'm *so* sorry."

No swearing or muttering. No recriminations.

We walked to the elevator together, with me in the lead.

"You changed your mind, Jamie. You're going to walk with me, huh? This should be fun."

"Yes, I need to do something to combat all the food I'm eating." He patted his belly.

I laughed, not sure that I believed him. I suspected he didn't want me walking alone.

As the cruise went on, I learned that Bobbie and Jamie wanted to protect me from any potential danger that lurked on board. So, in a united, military-like move, they flanked me, one ahead and one behind.

Each one had a particular style when giving directions.

Jamie gave commands like, "Go to the right, a little more, now straighten 'er out. You've got it. Good job!" When I walked with him, I felt as if I were learning to drive for the first time, with my cane as the stick shift. Jamie was patient, encouraging and specific. "That's a sharp turn. Now stop. Let's wait for Bobbie." His role was to keep us together, and he took it seriously.

Bobbie was more conversational and would interrupt herself to interject, "Go to the left—I mean the other left." Mixing up her rights and lefts always threw us into a fit of confusion and laughter. But she had a lot on her mind, like how others were reacting to my cane. She kept a running dialogue. "Those kids are like, 'Why does she get to play with a stick and we don't?' Do you see what a wide berth everyone gives you?"

I didn't really need any directions. My cane usually found the obstacles on its own. But the ship was crowded. Sometimes the passengers weren't paying attention, so Bobbie warned me before I hit them with my cane. I was used to walking fast and I had to remind myself to slow down. As for the reactions, I don't notice them anymore. I can't see facial expressions well and I'm far too focused on navigating my way around safely. I have adjusted to blocking out stares and comments.

Bobbie was quick to apologize to the other passengers if my cane nicked anyone passing by. She had a steady stream of comments like "Vision-impaired person coming through," or "Sorry, she didn't see you," that freed me up to use my cane without apology. I rather liked that.

When we reached Cape Canaveral a few days into the cruise, our group decided to head to Cocoa Beach instead. Bobbie called out, "Come on, Amy." I followed her voice and hurriedly explored the floor with my cane. "Whoa! I'm on the stairs, aren't I?" We had been using the elevator, so I didn't expect a flight of stairs. I laughed it off to soften her embarrassment about the near accident, which upset her. "Don't worry, my cane caught it," I said quickly.

We had a clown in the group who teased, "Way to go, Bobbie. Your grade just fell to a D."

"D! I got her up and down that tricky staircase last night, the one she was struggling with!"

"New day, new grade. Maybe if you try hard, she'll raise it…but only if you don't injure the instructor."

I guess they knew I used to teach.

I smiled so as not to draw any more attention to the incident. Bobbie had been trying hard, but people forget. Knowing where to draw the line between teasing and acceptance was like knowing the right dance moves. Being familiar with your partner made it easy, but dancing in a roomful of strangers made it difficult to predict each other's moves. I'm sure it felt like that to the group. I doubted any of them had been around a vision-impaired person before—let alone in tight quarters on a cruise ship—so I let them dance around me and did little to interfere.

After that, Bobbie shouted "Stairs!" every time we took them. I think that might become a code-word between us in the future to mean any kind of danger. It now makes us laugh.

When the group had booked the cruise, they had planned a kayaking excursion in the Bahamas. Bobbie, an experienced kayaker, couldn't wait for us to go out on the glass-bottomed kayak. She and I would man one together. I could hardly understand what one guide said until he suddenly enunciated clearly, "Important! If you see a fish, both of you in the kayak cannot lean out of the same side. It will tip over and that's the end of your fun."

He dramatically slapped his hands together. "It will be impossible for you to get in the kayak again. A guide will pick it up and you will have to come back onto the ferry."

I certainly had no desire to fall overboard in the Caribbean ocean.

The guide continued, "Male or female, the heavier one in each kayak goes in the back and paddles. The lighter one steers in front. Got it?"

I had to steer? I gulped. We were done for.

The five stairs leading to the bottom of the ferry and jumping-off place to the kayaks had Bobbie worried. "There's no railing, and you can't take your cane." The ferry shifted back and forth in the waves. "It's so unsteady…." Bobbie murmured.

Panicky shouts from the group unnerved me. "Someone stay with Amy! Don't let her go by herself! Make sure someone helps her!" I do best when others believe I can do whatever is expected. Their fears made me feel helpless and incapable.

They don't know what you can see, I coached myself. *You can handle this.*

The shouts seemed to rattle the guides too. It must have puzzled them why I needed special handling. After all, I didn't *look* blind and my cane was back at my seat. Everyone scrambled to get me down to the platform.

From the bottom of the ferry, the blurry ocean waves swelled as far as

I could see. My breath came faster. I could change my mind. I'd turn around and find a way to the steps. Rush back to my seat. Hold onto the safety rails with all my might. Yes, that's what I'd do.

"Jump!" one of the men shouted in heavily-accented English.

As my feet left the security of the ferry, several arms awkwardly reached out for me. I slipped through their grasp to land with an abrupt thump in the kayak. A large hand pushed me down roughly to the bottom, where the seat was supposedly located.

I made it! I wasn't bobbing around the ocean waves, ingesting salt water like I feared.

But I was in the back, not the front. Would we tip over?

"Hang on, here we go!" Bobbie said, suddenly self-assured and excited.

The choppy waves made me dizzy. The water glistened in a green sheen.

"Just relax," Bobbie said, "I'll steer us."

"But I'm supposed to paddle, right?"

"Don't worry. I got this."

My efforts were clumsy, but I didn't give up. It was important for me to do my part.

"Look at the fish below us. There's a blue striped one," Bobbie cried.

Looking through the glass-bottomed kayak was like looking through a television screen into a sometimes murky green lens. When I realized Bobbie had both the steering and paddling covered at the right times, I relaxed my grip on the paddles. The fear of me tipping the kayak gradually left. In its place, something much stronger washed over me. Exhilaration. Euphoria. I was doing something new and adventuresome.

Water slopped over the side of the kayak, and as I looked down, the water slapped my legs and feet.

"Are your feet getting wet?" Bobbie asked.

"Yep," I breathed. I was doing it. Not letting my fears get the better of me. Moving ahead in spite of them. Laughter bubbled up and surged through me as I half-heartedly navigated my paddle through the water.

I heard the kayakers shouting back and forth, "This fish swam right under my kayak! I swear it turned an eyeball up to me."

"No way! Cool. What did it look like?"

"Yellow with wide black and blue stripes. Gone now."

"Look at this one—skinny, just swam off the left side of the kayak."

"A whole school of something just passed by...."

There was a lull then someone shouted, "That's a...whaddatheycallit? Come on, help me."

"Dude, ya' gotta give us somethin' to go on...."

Their words were like the waves, lapping pleasantly around me as I peered through the green water in the glass-bottomed kayak, trying to glimpse even one exotic fish. But I never did. Maybe they darted away too fast or maybe my eyes couldn't pick up the details. It didn't matter. The tropical sun not only warmed my shoulders, it spread through me and seeped into my soul.

Bobbie made paddling seem easy. She looked so relaxed, even when we had to make our way around the bottleneck of snorkelers and kayakers. But she handled it effortlessly. I loved watching her in her element, totally confident and in charge.

We passed another kayak—the funny guy and Jamie. Bobbie called out, "Hi guys! Any cute fish your way?"

"Just the two in the boat," flirted the comedian.

Carefree moments like these pass too fast. This is how I will remember the Bahamas—warm sunshine, green water, laughter and wit among a circle of beautiful friends I've been privileged to become a part of—just *living* life. Perfection. When the guide called us in, our kayak returned last.

"See? You didn't tip the kayak over," my friend teased.

"Why would I do that? For the halibut?" I retorted.

Bobbie covered her mouth and nearly choked. "Amy, I'm going to tell your mother!"

Our lighthearted mood continued as we experienced water of another type on our return journey to the cruise ship. As the three of us dashed through the town in a tropical rainstorm, loud claps of thunder accompanied our footsteps.

We had planned to change our clothes and hit the bazaar near the harbor. I hoped this wasn't a game changer. I shouted over the pounding of the rain, "I used to work at Cedar Point, you know the amusement park in Sandusky, Ohio? When it rained, they made a killing on plastic rain ponchos. I betcha' they do something similar here," I said as persuasively as possible.

Leaving the cruise ship again, we spotted the ponchos. Bobbie's accommodating husband purchased one for each of the damsels. We were off on another adventure.

I turned to our souvenir hunting. This was my strength. Decades of practice had honed my skills. Over the years, friends had used me to help them reach the prices they wanted. I rubbed my hands together. Let the fun begin.

At the start, I was in my element. I bought a T-shirt and some traditional island dolls. Winding our way through the interior of the market, I found the fluctuations in lighting strained my eyes. I took off my sunglasses, hanging them on my shirt neck, and covered my bad eye in order to stop the blurring.

With his sonar tourist-spotting equipment, a dark-skinned vendor raced my way. "T-shirts. Any size."

"Turtle shell." A female vendor tugged on my arm. "Come look my children toy. Many you choose. You like name? I write."

Following the woman to her stand, I grinned. I knew the ropes. She just stole me away from another vendor. The woman gestured for me to choose from her large stand.

"Amy, these are so cute," Bobbie said.

The stand was in a dark corner and the heat started to bother me. "I can't see them," I said, eye fatigue making me tense. "What do they look like?" As I leaned in to better make out the variety of the small decorated shells hiding a spool of white string underneath, a strange thing happened. The paints blurred and the sizes seemed to shrink and swell. I bit my bottom lip to cover my confusion.

It's because I can't see them. I can't see them! Oh my gosh, I can't see them.

Tears stung my eyes.

"Can you…show me the…the red one?"

I could feel the woman's heavy breath on me as she leaned in closer. "Which one, dear?"

Claustrophobia set in. "Um, the blue, I mean a little boy's color. I want one for a toddler. Yes, my nephew." I tried to stop trembling.

She set the larger one down and handed me a smaller shell. "You want this one, dear?"

"Can you…describe it?" I'd never said that before.

The vendor named off various colors, which was nothing like seeing the patterns and designs on the actual toy. She set it on the ground and the contraption scuttled across the floor. She clapped her hands. "Beautiful, yes? You buy two."

"Let me hold it." Perhaps that would help me see it more clearly. I smoothed my hand over the shell. My voice grew more confident. "Yes, the name for this one is River. Write R-I-V-E-R on it, please." I jabbed at another one. "And on the red one, Gia. G-I-A."

After she finished, the vendor handed me the two toys.

In the light, I pulled the toys out of the bag to see them again. The bright colors came through. I suddenly realized I forgot to even bargain— for the first time ever. It would have been easy to let that get me down.

Bobbie took the blue toy from me and inspected it. "Amy, look at this!" She handed it to me.

RIVER was spelled R-I-L-E-Y.

It felt so good to laugh! That mistake lightened the mood again.

Every evening, the three of us went to the shows, which featured professional entertainers. My favorite was a bell-bottomed seventies evening of song and dance. Toward the end of the week, instead of the performance ending, the singers came out and the curtain closed behind them. While they sang "We Are Family," a stream of crew members filed onto the stage. I felt a lump fill my throat. These wonderful crew members who worked to make our cruise so enjoyable were indeed a family.

The recreational director proudly introduced the crew, including the Captain. I blinked back the tears. For me, it was not only a touching endorsement of the family atmosphere on the cruise, but also a poignant reminder of how much my own family had come together to make this trip possible for me—my nieces, brother-in-law and the friends and church members who offered to look in on my mom or cook dinner.

That evening, my mind flitted to the events of the past week—the morning walks, the sometimes comedic instructions that seemed to follow me everywhere, the moments of sharing our lives, and Bobbie's final words before falling asleep that night: "We are learning so much from you."

A truth dawned. Recalling how the waves sloshed over the sides of the kayak and onto my feet, that moment turned symbolic. I was getting my feet wet. It felt like a promise or a bridge to future travel. Like the murky green water beneath the boat, I couldn't see any details. But that didn't mean they wouldn't later make themselves clear.

I had managed to travel overseas with my mobility cane. I had done it and I could do it in the future, maybe next time with more independence.

My heart soared.

Navigating in tight straits is something I do every day of my life. It isn't a nuisance anymore because I need to do it to move forward. It's all a matter of perspective.

That little bit of insight instills fresh hope in me. I continue to grow every day. Lessons with my cane stretch me. They teach me to be open-minded, patient and positive, to appreciate the efforts of others and the here and now with my limited sight. Humor plays a role in every adventure.

Despite the dismal vision outlook destined for my future, with the help of my cane and friends, my life feels full of promise.

A NOTE TO READERS

If you're new to the world of vision loss, I feel for you. It overwhelms. It is easy to wonder how you will get through from one minute to the next hour, let alone the rest of your life. There are so many emotions to process. Like many things in life, ongoing vision loss happens in degrees, and acceptance comes gradually by seeking out help, guidance, tools, understanding and support. If this is where you're at, you might be interested in reading my first book, *Mobility Matters: Stepping Out in Faith*, where I share the story of how I came to terms with my vision loss through mobility training.

The seeds for *Cane Confessions* were the next step in my vision journey. They came from my blog posts, which made me realize how much my attitude affected my daily life in handling my vision loss and using my cane. A strong desire settled on my heart to encourage others who struggle with the emotions that go along with choosing to use a cane. I also wanted to educate those who don't understand the real and imagined struggles a cane creates for a vision-impaired individual, and, specifically, what living with the inconsistencies of RP is like.

These stories don't exist to say life is going to fall into place and you will figure out the answers you need in order to fit into some kind of meaningful group—at whatever degree of blindness you face. I've compiled my experiences to say it's possible to choose joy, humor and understanding in spite of the insecurities that go along with progressive vision loss.

The hope close to my heart is for you to put on strong binoculars that allow you to focus on the good that surrounds the messiness daily life challenges us all with.

Most of the insights I've gleaned from my experiences in *Cane Confessions* come from actually writing them down and pondering what I've learned. My belief is that nothing is wasted if we can glean truths from our vulnerabilities and share lessons that help us all move forward to understand each other better.

With much love and gratitude to all my readers.

Amy

CONTACT THE AUTHOR

Thank you so much for reading my book. I'd greatly appreciate it if you could post a quick review on Amazon please.

I hope you'll join my mailing list (http://eepurl.com/1682P) to receive some bonus stories about my chaotic adventures and be amongst the first to hear when my next book is released.

I'd love to hear your feedback on *Cane Confessions* and am happy to answer any questions you may have, so do please get in touch with me by:

- emailing me: abovaird@verizon.net
- viewing my website: www.amybovaird.com
- following me on social media:
  - Twitter: @amy_bovaird
  - Facebook: amybovairdauthor
  - Pinterest: amybovairdautho/
  - LinkedIn: amy-bovaird-157bb420

I hope you will read my memoir *Mobility Matters: Stepping Out in Faith* which follows my journey as an international teacher into the acceptance that I am now losing my eyesight.

If you like memoirs, I recommend you pop over to Facebook group We Love Memoirs to chat with me and other authors there.

I look forward to hearing from you.

Amy

ACKNOWLEDGEMENTS

Without the following influences and dedicated support in my life, you wouldn't be reading this book. I am so grateful to:

God—who planted both the seed for this book through my blog posts and the right people in my life to bring it to fruition.

My mother—for being patient about my long hours on the computer, and *my brother*, for all the speaking engagements he has taken me to in order to share my first book while I was writing my second.

Kathy, Sue, Lynn, James, Bettie-Lou and Crystal—friends from near and far who cheered me on (and did some shaming when I needed a kick in the pants to reach the next milestone.) We all need friends to bring the best out in us.

Judie Gleason—my business-savvy driver and friend who journeyed down the author road with me.

Jennifer Brownlee—small business mentor who helped navigate the business side of my author journey.

My friends—who lived these experiences with me and helped me glean insights. You know who you are.

Melissa and Larry Beahm—a dynamic husband and wife musical duo and creators of my children's song, "The White Cane Song." They spread my optimistic message and, as they travel and perform across the United States, help change perceptions of blind people.

My Facebook Cane Confession *prayer warriors*—a group of seventeen Christ-centered people who faithfully prayed for my needs and progress in my writing ministry whenever I posted a request.

Aldine Hecker—my biggest fan. She prayed me safely through my travels overseas through lean financial times and has promoted me and my writing for over thirty years.

RJ Thesman—my patient editor, who coached me through the pages of this book and brought clarity to my experiences.

Pennwriters Critique Groups—talented members who helped me hone my writing craft and dig deeper into my emotions, also ensuring that I made what I didn't see, clear to my readers. Thank you!

Maribel Steel—Author, editor and role model who has turned her own blindness into an art form, impacting my attitude and optimism.

West County Lions Club—its members supported progress as I completed new chapters of my book. A special shout-out to *Margaret and*

John Dudkowski, Dr. Katie Kutterna and Marty Heid who ensured I had transportation to my weekly critique group.

Ant Press—Victoria Twead and Jacky Donovan. I can't thank Ant Press enough for taking on *Cane Confessions* and believing in my message.

Bernadette Harrison—professional artist and illustrator and a close first cousin on my father's side of the family. We always talked 'one day' of collaborating together on a book. That day has finally come and our work together makes this book even more special to me.

Heather Lamison Desuta—the book designer who, in short order, put her skills to good use and made my overall book cover look compelling.

Rebecca Widdecombe—a hometown fan, so grateful for our friendship, for her sharing my books with others and touting my speaking talents.

Katharine Godbey—my helpful web technician who keeps my website and blog up and running.

Diana Starrett and *Matt Harris*—for their long-distance support as I fleshed out my experiences in this book.

And last, but by no means least, my readers—without you, my books would have no purpose. I'm so grateful. Please keep reading and passing on my message of optimism.

ANT PRESS BOOKS

If you enjoyed this book, you may also enjoy these titles:

MEMOIRS

Chickens, Mules and Two Old Fools by Victoria Twead (Wall Street Journal Top 10 bestseller)

Two Old Fools ~ Olé! by Victoria Twead

Two Old Fools on a Camel by Victoria Twead (New York Times bestseller x 3)

Two Old Fools in Spain Again by Victoria Twead

One Young Fool in Dorset (The Prequel) by Victoria Twead

One Young Fool in South Africa (The Prequel) by Joe and Victoria Twead

How not to be a Soldier: My Antics in the British Army by Lorna McCann

Heartprints of Africa: A Family's Story of Faith, Love, Adventure, and Turmoil by Cinda Adams Brooks

Simon Ships Out: How One Brave, Stray Cat Became a Worldwide Hero by Jacky Donovan

Seacat Simon: The Little Cat Who Became a Big Hero (children's version of the above book for age 8 to 11)

Smoky: How a Tiny Yorkshire Terrier Became a World War II American Army Hero, Therapy Dog and Hollywood Star by Jacky Donovan

Instant Whips and Dream Toppings: A True-Life Dom Rom Com by Jacky Donovan

Fat Dogs and French Estates ~ Part I by Beth Haslam

Fat Dogs and French Estates ~ Part II by Beth Haslam

Into Africa with 3 Kids, 13 Crates and a Husband by Ann Patras

More Into Africa with 3 Kids, some Dogs and a Husband by Ann Patras

Midwife: A Calling by Peggy Vincent
Midwife: A Journey by Peggy Vincent

Serving is a Pilgrimage by John S. Basham

Moment of Surrender: My Journey Through Prescription Drug Addiction to Hope and Renewal by Pj Laube

Horizon Fever — Explorer A E Filby's own account of his extraordinary expedition through Africa, 1931 – 1935 by A E Filby

One of its Legs are Both the Same by Mike Cavanagh

FICTION

A is for Abigail by Victoria Twead (Sixpenny Cross 1)
B is for Bella by Victoria Twead (Sixpenny Cross 2)

Parched by Andrew C. Branham (Parched Series 1)

CHILDREN'S BOOKS

Seacat Simon: The Little Cat Who Became a Big Hero (age 8 to 11) by Jacky Donovan

The Rise of Agnil by Susan Navas (Agnil's World 1)
Agnil and the Wizard's Orb by Susan Navas (Agnil's World 2)
Agnil and the Tree Spirits by Susan Navas (Agnil's World 3)
Agnil and the Centaur's Secret by Susan Navas (Agnil's World 4)

Morgan and the Martians by Victoria Twead

NON FICTION

How to Write a Bestselling Memoir: Three Steps — Write, Publish, Promote by Victoria Twead

ABOUT THE AUTHOR

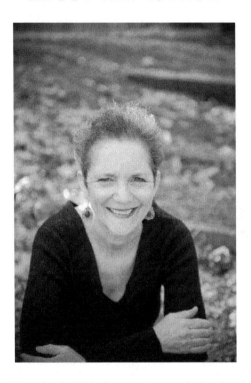

Amy is a vision-impaired Christian author and speaker. Diagnosed with Retinitis Pigmentosa at the age of 28, she later discovered it was part of an even rarer hereditary disease called Usher Syndrome, the leading cause of deaf blindness in the world. To date, there is no cure.

Having taught in Latin America, South East Asia and the Middle East, Amy often features glimpses of these and other cultures in her writing.

She went from riding in and on top of buses in Latin America to catching the subway and trains in the Far East, not to mention *bajajs, becaks* and *bemos* and even a water buffalo on the backroads of West Sumatra, and then on to 4x4s and camels in the Middle East. Now her travel is accompanied by a simple cane but with no less enthusiasm.

Amy blogs about the challenges she faces as she loses more vision and hearing, but more importantly, she shares the lessons God reveals to her through her difficulties. You can read about her experiences on her blog—www.amybovaird.com.